Written with charm and grace, this refreshing book reminds us that food isn't what feeds us, but that communion with others and with the inner life is the real food of substance. Our lives are the treat, not what we crave at the dinner table.

~G. Miki Hayden, author

"*Release Your Obsession with Cheat DAZE: Heal from the Inside Out*...is such a relatable read! The personal experience coupled with reasonable application is a much needed journey to recovery."

~Leah Jordan Meahl, Author of *The Threshold*

Release Your Obsession with Cheat DAZE will resonate with anyone seeking a path to true emotional freedom from food. In this impactful book, Dr. Ortigara Crego provides a perspective and road map for that power, combining inspiring real-life stories with practical examples and tools. This is wonderful book with a powerful message and beautiful vision on how to heal from the inside out—one person at a time.

~Dara Bushman, Psy.D., A Licensed Clinical Psychologist in recovery from food addiction; practices as a specialist in eating disorders.

In *Release Your Obsession with Cheat DAZE: Heal from the Inside Out*; Dr. Lisa Ortigara once again introduces the would-be dieter to what they really need: a complete lifestyle change. As Dr. Ortigara Crego so eloquently points out, "When your diet is cleared of toxic foods, you'll want to eat foods that are clean and real." And she couldn't be more right! I know from personal experience that once you switch to real, whole foods, you will no longer crave processed junk. Nature holds a bounty of flavors to satisfy our palettes, which unfortunately have been dulled by the deluge of high fructose corn syrup and chemicals in the plastic-like "food" that makes up the standard American Diet (as referenced in this wonderful book".

I especially enjoyed Dr. Ortigara Crego's account of how food addiction causes its sufferers to lose control with a single "cheat' and how this turns into a cheat daze, as this is not something us non-food addicts generally "get", but the way the information is presented here really helped me understand what a lot of my peers are going through.

Another favorite is how the author weaves in spiritual needs and the connection between feeding the belly and the soul. I highly recommend this book to anyone who is struggling with dieting and food obsession/addiction (and friends and family struggling to understand what the food addict is going through). The personal inventory questions are invaluable and Dr. Ortigara Crego's lifestyle changes provide a simple blueprint to get healthy and stay that way once and for all.

~Riya Anne Polcastro, *Author of Death by Gluten: How Undiagnosed Celiac Almost Cost Me My Life.*

Release Your Obsession with Cheat DAZE

Heal from the Inside Out

Dr. Lisa M. Ortigara Crego

Release Your Obsession with Cheat DAZE: Heal from the Inside Out

ISBN: 978-0-9993025-2-1
Library of Congress Control Number: 2019950648

The author of this book does not dispense medical advice or prescribe the use of any technique as a form of treatment for physical, emotional, or medical problems without the advice of a physician, either directly or indirectly. The intent of the author is only to offer information of a general nature to help you in your quest for emotional, spiritual, and physical well-being. In the event you use any of the information in this book for yourself, which is your constitutional right, the author and the publisher assume no responsibility for your actions.

Madeira Publishing
Hollywood, Florida
Madeirapublising.com

MEDICAL DISCLAIMER

The information presented in this book is the result of twenty-plus years of practice experience and observational research by the author. The author of this book does not dispense medical advice or prescribe the use of any technique as a form of treatment for physical, emotional, or medical problems without the advice of physician, either directly or indirectly. The information in this book, by necessity, is of a general nature and not a substitute for an evaluation or treatment by a competent medical and psychological specialist. If you believe you are in need of medical or psychological intervention, please see a medical and/or psychological practitioner as soon as possible. The stories in this book are true. The names and circumstances of the stories have been changed to protect the anonymity of patients. The intent of the author is only to offer information of a general nature to help you in your quest for emotional, spiritual, and physical wellbeing. In the event you use any of the information in this book for yourself, which is your constitutional right, the author and the publisher assume no responsibility for your actions.

Dedicated to my husband, Joseph Vincent Crego,
for his unfailing positivity throughout our marriage.
My I-want-it-all attitude and proactive mindset
stem from his unwavering belief in me,
and his support of my journey.
I love you, Joe.

Foreword

Do you eat healthy until it comes to weekends, vacations, holidays, and parties? You're not alone. Millions of us have struggled with these "cheat days," only to reap the consequences, which are never worth the indulgence.

In *Release Your Obsession with Cheat DAZE: Heal from the Inside Out*, Dr. Lisa Ortigara Crego focuses on developing constructive relationships with food, body, and lifestyle, long-term. By emphasizing the event and the people connection rather than the food, she encourages self-confidence, self-love, and a positive attitude, shedding any feelings of shame, blame, and deprivation. Each chapter begins with a carefully selected quotation to inspire. In her words, "You can eat clean no matter where you are, or what's going on—and not feel short changed."

Having read both of her previous books, *Release Your Obsession with Food: Heal from the Inside Out* and *Release Your Obsession with Diet Chatter: Heal from the Inside Out*, I had become familiar with her philosophies and believed in her viewpoint of accepting healthy eating as a lifestyle and not a diet. Her impressive credentials as a clinical psychotherapist, addiction psychologist, and visiting professor, as well as her over 25 years treating patients in clinical private practice in the field of eating disorders, qualify her as an expert in writing about recovery from food addiction and eating disorders.

Quoting researched articles to validate her points and interspersing experiences of her own and real stories of the clients she has treated, she accentuates the above themes in this life-changing book.

Maintaining that food is not the chief happening, and that you can "eat your way through any place, event, or situation—no matter what, or where you are," she shows us how this can be possible in a chapter about her personal travel in Europe. I was particularly interested, since I could never bring myself to forgo the pasta, pizza, and gelato on my frequent trips to my beloved Italy as a travel blogger. But on my latest overseas expedition to London and other parts of the UK, armed with what I've learned, I stayed away from sugar, flour, and wheat without feeling swindled, and came home three pounds lighter. Her words, "embrace the moment, not the food," rang true. I can't wait for my next Italy trip when I plan to follow the healthy lifestyle I've adopted due to Dr. Lisa's influence. It's the change in lifestyle, rather than a diet that "allows our commitment to last a lifetime."

Dr. Lisa shows us how to be free in regard to our consumption and able to enjoy a wide variety of foods, fresh, non-processed, and healthy. By encouraging us to visualize what we want and believe it, she shows us how to eradicate the obsessions surrounding eating.

Dr. Lisa's argument from the biochemical point of view is a strong one—the same reward- and pleasure-centers in the brain triggered by addictive drugs like cocaine are also activated by foods, especially sugar, fat, and salt, and trigger brain chemicals such as dopamine, to make us feel good.

As an added benefit, Dr. Lisa includes practical tips and recipes, like raspberry pancakes and raspberry coffee ice cream, or chocolate pineapple ice cream. Included at the end of each chapter are personal inventory questions for each of us to answer.

Anyone facing the struggles of cheat days in food choices will find this book truly transforming. I can't recommend it enough! It has changed my life in more ways than I thought possible. "Life and happiness are about now…not tomorrow, and not yesterday." I consider this quote of hers to be most inspiring.

Margie Miklas, author of *My Amalfi Coast Love Affair*

Introduction

Do not go where the path may lead,
go instead where there is no path
and leave a trail.
~Ralph Waldo Emerson

I'll never forget the moment my mom said to me, "Lisa, I think you have an eating disorder." I was astounded that she had just realized this fact—especially since at the time, I was in the process of recovery after years and years of struggles with binge eating and bulimia through over-exercising. I was about thirty-seven years old. The topic came up because we were gathered in the kitchen at her Tampa Bay home in Florida, where mom was preparing a lovely roasted chicken with roasted potatoes while I was tending to the salad, chopping juicy red cherry tomatoes, crisp cucumbers, and sweet onions, all mixed in with romaine lettuce for a succulent dinner we would soon share.

At one point, Mom began cutting huge chunks of butter, placing them strategically over every piece of chicken, making sure she covered each spot, not to mention freely pouring olive oil over the potatoes. At this stage, I said, "Whoa, Mom, what are you doing? That's a boatload of fat you just plastered all over that chicken!" And right then she looked me straight in the eyes, and firmly said that maybe I had an eating disorder. *What? You are just now realizing this?*

The funny thing was all those years of my obsessively eating copious amounts of junk food on my cheat day(s), inhaling as fast as I could, she never said a word—and now here I was eating more healthfully than I'd ever done in my life, and she began to take note and make known that she thought I was being a bit fixated. *How ironic.*

On this very day in the kitchen with Mom I had my eyes open about me, my mother, and even my grandmother, who we then proceeded to talk about. Ma, my mom's mom, Ruth, who'd been in a nursing home at the end of her life, changed from a very ornery, difficult woman to a kind human being. We arrived on the topic of my grandmother because my mom also noted I was a bit kinder and easier as of late. She wondered if something was going on for such a change. Normally, I was irritable and difficult.

We began to talk about my healthy lifestyle of eating natural foods at regular intervals in right portions and balance, coupled with moderate daily exercise, which catapulted my change—not to mention a hundred-pound weight loss.

At that moment in the kitchen, I had the revelation that my grandmother became so sweet when the white habit nuns who ran the nursing home out in the country in Wisconsin fed her natural foods and put love birds in her room to sing to her, while she practiced simple living. I compared myself to her, as I too became gentler and more soft spoken after turning to unprocessed foods, letting go of sugar, flour, and wheat.

My mother and I went on to discuss the money habits of my grandmother and of my mother as well. I was dirt poor at the time and watched money slip through my grandmother's hand as if she were trying to hold sand while each granule slipped from her fingers. She went from riches to rags to riches to rags. My mother also had poor money-management skills. I was in debt up to my eyeballs.

After that kitchen episode, I began to unravel the connection between managing money and food, and sprinkling in self-love and self-care, all of which were partial solutions to releasing obsessions so that I could heal from the inside out.

Ma was NOT the sweet, loveable grandma we all wish for—you know the one who puts out cookies and milk. No, she was mean, and definitely had it in for me. She didn't like me—as you'll read farther down when I tell My Story. My grandmother went through hundreds of thousands of dollars, spending on this and that, not knowing how to save; eating and drinking whatever she wanted; sporting extra weight to prove it; and at the end of her life had no money, was overweight and in very poor health, not living her best life—*but she did become sweet.*

No, that was not going to be me, to have a change in my mid-eighties. NO, I thought at that very moment, leaning over the counter chopping onions, tomatoes, cucumbers, and romaine—and I'm hoping this is not going to be you. It's time to practice self-love, to live within your means, and to move away from the standard American diet (SAD) of processed foods—SAD indeed. The time has come to eat healthfully, no matter where you are or who you're with, and most of all to be happy, healthy, and wise.

I began to invest time in reading how to become debt free with books such as Dave Ramsey's *The Total Money Makeover*, *Think and Grow Rich* by Napoleon Hill, and *Don't Worry, Make Money* by Richard Carlson, along with healthy lifestyle books such as *Food and Mood,* and later, *Eat Your Way to Happiness*, both penned by popular dietitian Elizabeth Somer. I then watched my life turn around as self-care took over, and I began to live debt free and toxic food free. You can too. You can celebrate ***all*** of life's festivities without cheat-day mentality, stay on track with healthy foods, and not feel deprived, while simultaneously leaving behind the shame, blame, and self-judgment.

More than twenty-five years after that kitchen conversation with my mother, I'm privileged to make my living teaching thousands of people—men and women, young and old—how to live their best lives through self-love, self-care, eating real foods, living within their means, and abandoning the SAD way the majority of people are trying to nourish themselves. Now I'm happy to report that when you strip away all the processed foods; learn how to eat whole, rich foods with nutrients; and spend on quality foods rather than fast foods, you will have an abundance of money to travel and see the world and eat without a food-fester, cheat-day mentality. I promise.

I've helped patients and readers alike, and now I'd like to help you live free.

Imagine

Merrily free. Stop and envision what you would feel like being at peace from the cheat day mentality—that for once you have no urge to eat everything and anything once a week, or before your tomorrow diet promise kicks in. What would you feel like going anywhere at any time with anyone, harboring no worries about gaining weight or losing control with food—or better yet being satisfied with exactly who you are, as you are. To no longer use food as treats, rewards, bargaining chips, or as an indulgence of whatever you want one day a week—or whatever deal you've made with yourself.

Imagine it's your birthday, Christmas, Chanukah, a long holiday weekend or that you're somewhere in Italy wandering the streets with all kinds of tantalizing aromas whirling around in the air, but you're okay—no more cheat day food frenzy, "gotta have it" kind of attitude. No more, "if I just lost x-number of pounds…"

What would you feel like waking up day after day, any place at any time in your life, and eating "normal" with no head talk and no guilt and no cravings—being perfectly aligned with a healthy way of eating, no matter where you are, who you're with, or what's going on in your life. And imagine further that you feel no gripping "will power" or guilt, or jonsing or any of those other old familiar feelings when that *feeling* comes on and you know you're going to cave.

No, this book is not like the common diet book—it's not about a diet at all—it's on the subject of a freedom you never imagined—freedom from the *Cheat DAZE*, food frenzy that seizes you on any and every *special* occasion. Well, no more. This is a new way of relating to food.

Accept that all of that is possible.

The Promise

No book, psychologist, psychotherapist, spiritualist, or life coach, can guarantee that out-of-control eating during every function in any given situation will cease for the rest of your life, or that you will embrace food-fest-frenzy relief without a taint, just as no one can guarantee you will be financially secure for the remainder of your life after playing Power Ball and winning millions of dollars—or that you will live life in perfect harmony every single minute of your life without a blemish—even if you live in the best of situations.

But I can promise to show you ways to maneuver through life's festivities at peace with food and all that such relaxation entails, if you practice the suggestions laid out in this book. As you power through these pages, you will master traveling, long weekends, holidays, birthdays, Memorial and Labor Day, and yes, even funerals, with your food selection that fits your healthy lifestyle—and no more "just this one time" attitude.

By the time you finish reading ***Release Your Obsession with Cheat DAZE: Heal from the Inside Out***, you will be able to skillfully arrest any inner and outer turmoil focused on the one cheat day—that often turns into days—and the DAZE, as you enter zombie zone. But instead, for once, you will live free from the burdens and fears of caving into sugary, high-fat food selections, no longer white knuckling and forcing change in an unnatural way. You will no longer live for the cheat day. You will have collected an arsenal of strategies to silence the planned temptations, and once and for all free yourself from the burdens you have entrapped in your food fests frenzy, any celebration *must-eat* mentality.

My Start

Very often, the work we choose in order to make a living stems from deep-seated personal experiences. When I was just a small child I was attracted to sugar-laden foods and preferred them to any kind of nutritional "real" food. I was *that kid* who preferred to eat sweet, sticky foods to any remotely real food. I was that kid who had temper tantrums, lying on the floor kicking and screaming, red faced, temples bulging from an out-and-out rage, screaming, "I DON'T WANT THAT FOOD. I WANT CANDY—I HATE THAT. DON'T MAKE ME EAT IT…I HATE YOU!"

In first grade, a stick-thin girl with long, stringy, unwashed hair named Karen B. sat across from me in the lunchroom, plates and forks clinking and clashing, a watered-down casserole smelling of dirty-sock aroma wafting in the air, as each snot-nosed kid scarfed the servings placed before them under the nun's watchful eye, as no food was to go uneaten.

On this particular day, Karen's nose was leaking beyond her control, soaked up with any napkin she could get her hands on, and at some point after coveting mine, to no avail, she reverted to using the back of her hand to wipe each drop. My stomach churned and revolted. I couldn't eat.

From that day forward, the lunchroom was my personal battle zone where I easily became turned off to food. When I could, I toted my own meal from home, insisting on chocolate milk, cookies, and anything that didn't look like real food. If I was forced to eat the lunches, I got creative, hiding inedibles under my napkin or accidentally dropping a good portion on the floor.

You see, the nuns, in their black habits trimmed in white, with long, chunky rosaries wrapped around their waists (hanging length-wise down their gowns and clinking as the two on patrol stood in military position between two oversized, dark matte-green garbage cans), were lifting napkins and poking around the students' plates with long, wooden pointers, insuring we ate every bite so that no child *out there* would be left unfed. Meanwhile, the stench of decaying foods swirled in the air.

I evolved as a sneaking, food-hiding kid. *Let the festivities begin…*

I recall when I first began to experience food fests frenzy in any type of celebratory situation (or not). My behavior went undetected because I was one of those skinny kids. Between Mom and the nuns at school, I was assigned to be part of the *clean plate* club, meaning I was not to leave leftovers as children somewhere were starving. Where, I hadn't a clue, nor who or in what country these kids were, or if they even really existed.

All I knew was I didn't want to eat the slop they pushed on me. So, instead, I snuck and stole and hid foods—undetected. As part of all this choreography around food, I seemed to feel I had the green light to eat all I wanted on my birthday, vacations, long weekends—oh heck simply passing a two-day weekend warranted a food fest of some sort *until I began to get fat.*

Once my body and mind brought me to the out-of control place, sheer panic took hold. Though terrified, I decided any event was a reason to eat out of control, with the plan of "fixing" my slip-ups after the occasion passed. Even my greatest and gravest attempts afterward, though, didn't work because I didn't understand how to change my relationship with food.

My full-blown eating disorder appeared at my tail end of twelve, budding on thirteen, years of age.

Your Opportunity

My journey and recovery from food fests frenzy, obsession with food, and mind-poison chatter and commotion without interruption eventually led to the awakening of my passion to counsel others. I wanted to help those suffering from eating issues and faulty thinking, both of which mess with our natural happy buttons concerning food.

After watching countless patients learn to quiet their obsession with cheat day mentality coupled with diet mindset, I knew with certainty that this chaotic on-and-off behavior can be superseded by productive, healthy food choices without crippling a trip or festive occasion.

I have seen, without a doubt, that dialing down the food-centered arguments in the head can be achieved by making conscious, healthy food choices without losing the ambience and fun on any trip, holiday, or festive occasion, not to mention the sad times when a loss is followed by a celebration of life, including foods to comfort the soul.

I learned this firsthand, and now I'm passing my understanding on to you.

My goal for you is to live a contented life without disruptive cheat days.

Release Your Obsession with Cheat DAZE: Heal from the Inside Out is for anyone trying to end the vicious cycle of continuous on-and-off dieting, especially surrounding festive occasions and long weekends. This is most definitely not a diet book or a get-skinny-quick kind of offering. That would be suggesting some sort of fad diet, which only enhances the chaotic diet behavior.

My goal is to free you. As Ralph Waldo Emerson states: "Do not go where the path may lead, go instead where there is no path and leave a trail." The path of setting up planned cheat days will lead you into the food fest abyss; go instead where no path exists and make *your* trail. My goal is to suggest a trail for you to create and for once release your obsession with cheat DAZE, food fests frenzy. Rest assured that while this is no easy task, it is definitely achievable.

My first book from the Release Your Obsession series, ***Release Your Obsession with Food,*** addresses food addiction and how to tame the giant within. My second book, ***Release Your Obsession with Diet Chatter,*** addresses the inner voice that at times is loud and disruptive, while at other times only a soft whisper—and at still other times, barely audible. But the voice is there…and it's trying to take hold of you every chance it gets.

This latest book builds off of releasing your obsession with food and with diet chatter, so you can ***Release Your Obsession with Cheat DAZE*** mentality, the food festivity frenzy, where you gorge yourself on the "forbidden foods" for one day—at least. Instead, I will lead you to heal from the inside out.

I don't have to teach the cheat day concept to you, or try to help you "get it," because if you picked up this book, you already know food addiction and the inner chatter, and all-out binge wars at every occasion including long weekends because the urge to cheat has hung around you for a long, long time—almost teasing you as if it were your friend.

This is no friend.

This is destruction.

Both obsessive eating and taunting thinking move you as far away as possible from any Divine Source, Love, or spiritual awakening, or whatever you want to label it. And now, we want to kick the cheat day mentality to the curb so you can truly be free in Italy, Ireland, India, Indiana, Wisconsin, or anywhere you please during any festivity or occasion.

Let me show you the way…

In my earliest book, ***Release Your Obsession with Food: Heal from the Inside Out,*** my goal was to present a rich and provocative understanding of chemical imbalance, psychology, and spirituality—a bio-psycho-spiritual point of view, as it relates to compulsive eating.

And I also intended my second book, ***Release Your Obsession with Diet Chatter: Heal from the Inside Out***, to present a multi-layered and challenging understanding of chemical imbalance, psychology, and spirituality—also taking a bio-psycho-spiritual point of view, not as it relates to compulsive eating but rather to dig deeper into our obsessive negative mind talk about our bodies and the way we hope to use fad diets to become skinny—resulting in a constant murmur of dialogue nagging in our thoughts.

Release Your Obsession with Cheat DAZE: Heal from the Inside Out is no different than the first two books in that we are again looking through a bio-psycho-spiritual lens, but will work in conjunction with the first two because you are now armed and ready to take on the world.

Kinsey's Self-War

A recent patient I'll call Kinsey, whose concerns I didn't know yet, began to express her attachment to sugar—that she wanted to control it and be able to eat it in moderation. As she was laying out her story, she began twisting her interlocked fingers then leaned forward and looked at me intensely with her fiery black eyes. Her jaw tight, she said, "I can't imagine going home to my country and not eating my specialty foods." She stated this so powerfully the impact was as if someone had died.

Tears cascading down her cheeks, she proceeded to tell me that all festive occasions are tied to food, together with her feelings—all rolled into one. She didn't know how to separate one from the other. In other words, the only way to have a real vacation experience or a family connection or enjoy the moment was if she ate specified foods connected to each event. Having a trip home without those foods she grew up on was impossible—yet when she ate them, she felt shame, blame, and self-judgment. Kinsey was at war with herself.

And Kinsey signed up for cheat day mentality when she returned to her homeland: Panama.

Kinsey is not alone. Somehow food and feelings are inseparable and become the fun. But occasions are not only about the food. They're about the people and the connection to those people. Celebrations are about the experience, the memories you're creating. The event is NOT about the sugar-laden concoction your Aunty Leslie made—it's about Aunt Lesley.

As in ***Release Your Obsession with Food*** and ***Release Your Obsession with Diet Chatter,*** the focus in ***Release Your Obsession with Cheat DAZE*** is on spiritual recovery, eating natural whole foods, and instruction as to how to stop the insane fixation on vacation foods, or *time off,* meaning food fest, party-down time. The key word is fest. Something clicks and connects food festers to any festivity that warrants eating everything you haven't eaten in a while or the usually forbidden foods—or somehow you'll miss out on the event if you don't pile your plate high with rich, non-nutrient foods that hold some meaning from long ago.

Explorations

I have set up this book to take you through a series of explorations, just the way I would if you came to me weekly as a private patient for psychotherapy, sharing positive and negative experiences from my own life and the lives of others who walked this path prior to, during, and after recovery. The book opens with a discussion and understanding of ***Cheat DAZE—The Food Frenzy***, unpacking the *what* and *why* as it's wrapped around ***cheat day*** mentality.

My goal is to show you how to release obsessive, negative, self-destructive food and festivity connections and build a confident self on all occasions whether food is involved or not. My goal is to remove the food-as-the-center-of-your-universe attitude and replace it with food as your lifeline but not your entertainment.

Along with an attempt to reveal how I have come to grips with the incessant *party-down* mentality, I also endeavor to help readers meet this difficult challenge through practical, structured, step-by-step, synthesized information and advice, including anecdotes to demonstrate how individuals may obtain relief and resolution of never-ending issues arising from destructive behavior as it relates to any festivity eating.

As you weave through the chapters, you will encounter discussions as to why the food fests with the intention of a cheat day become your primary focus rather than the event itself. Why downtime leads to food partying. And you'll be led to examine how the food giant takes up residence in your activities while your diet mentality remains intact afterward. A book on *Cheat Daze* that show up as food fest frenzies would be missing the mark if the topics of certain food behaviors were ignored, such as: getaways to indulge; cruising open waters with vats of foods at your beck and call; fun seen through the lens of diet mentality; and weekend warrior attitude—or any celebration conduct centering on food for that matter.

Realignment from loss of a loved one to what's eating you while diving into a holiday fog and food addiction laced with sugar, salt, and fat attachment takes front and center first—where we power through understanding how the gooey attraction of certain "treats" took up residence in your ever-food-fan affair, anyway.

Working through and realigning using a bag of tools such as learning a new relationship with foods, understanding how to put together a healthy food shopping list, and how to maneuver through grocery stores spills over from one chapter to the next, giving you the control and expertise you need for when you aren't in the comfort of your usual environment. How, you ask? First you must start from where you are, and then as you venture out to parties and trips away from your town, city, state, and even country, you will be a pro at handling all situations.

As you become more at ease, you will handle the twists and turns of life during out-of–the-country excursions, embarking on would-be cruise frenzies, and yes, even on your birthday.

The chapters also unpack the importance of understanding and employing each tool on the journey of recovery from obsessive, inner, negative conversations such as, "but it's my birthday," or an "I will miss out if I don't eat this or taste that" kind of thought process.

As you ***Turn the Corner***, food and mood and the sacred art of mealtime and preparations of meals takes hold. A continuous consideration of linking your efforts with your own unique understanding of a Higher Source, relationships, and food is intertwined and threaded throughout the pages. In addition, you'll find the chapters speckled with words of self-care and self-love, moving away from excessive spending of hard-earned money to maintain a standard American diet, which is both sad and costly, to a healthful American diet wherein you spend less money eating better quality foods.

I'd like to think that everyone has a personal take on his or her own *Divine Source*, whether from Judaism, for instance, or through Buddhism, Sikhism, Christianity, or whatever reference point, perhaps combined with that or another particular spiritual training.

Regardless of *your* concept of Source, you can tap into your own heart and soul using the approach that fits your belief system best, to find an authentic foundation and open the door to a much deeper, more soulful experience of life.

And of course, we will examine working through the emotional component that comes with the promise of a *cheat day* as we turn another year older, and how that can be rerouted to gratitude for breath and appreciation for the role of food in our lives. We will look at how every day can be a good day, from the gathering of food in the supermarket to sitting down at your table embracing the sacred art of mealtime—whether here or traipsing through Italy. All pathways to releasing your obsessions with cheat days and food fest frenzy ideology are incorporated into this book.

If you will examine your personal inventory as questions appear following each chapter and practice the golden nuggets scattered throughout the pages, by the time you reach the end of this material, you will have begun to change your life.

My immediate goal is to help you release your obsession with the food fest frenzy ideation and connection in twenty-one days or less, thanks to:

- ✓ The book's groundbreaking identification of the *what* and the *why* of believing *food* is the event—that food will *complete* you.
- ✓ The incorporation of easy, step-by-step customizable day-to-day "outpatient" actions to help you navigate through the jungle of temptations and old belief systems from childhood or cultural connections.
- ✓ Personal Inventory Questions throughout, designed to identify and reprogram your cheat day mentality and open your unique natural/spiritual path to recovery.

My suggestion is that you first read through the book once to orient yourself to this approach. Then you can slowly read the book again—only this time working through the questions following the end of each chapter.

As you read, you'll also note that every chapter opens with an inspirational quote from a spiritual leader, author, or the Bible. Don't skip these valuable morsels of wisdom, as they're real treasures, designed to start you thinking at a deeper level.

To help the reader best use ***Release Your Obsession with Cheat DAZE: Heal from the Inside Out***, the book is organized into three basic parts.

The first section *(Cheat DAZE—The Food Frenzy)* explores the obsession with the idea that food will complete you. Yes, it keeps you alive and is a necessity and should be enjoyed, but it's not entertainment. I follow the inner workings and trappings of diet mentality prior to the *what and whys* of food frenzy here with a clear explanation of emotional attachment and romancing holidays, vacations, and celebrations, and the cultural connections ending with any excuse to eat. My goal is to analyze the effect and impact of food festivity thinking while unmasking the role of the emotional connection to food, with the ultimate intention of changing your attitude and thoughts about food, leading to recovery.

The second section (*Realignment*) takes you from out-of-control cheat day food frenzy celebrations to understanding how food addiction, or possibly eating disorders, may play a role in your thought processes and attachment to sugar, salt, and fat. Alignment is only possible if you can move through the grocery store aisles with confidence, knowing you can create lovely, wholesome dishes for yourself, your family, and guests at parties you may hold in your home. You will find that the grocery store is not the big, bad giant you might have imagined it to be but rather your opportunity to fill your home with luscious, edible, healthful and even healing foods that are delicious yet nutritious.

You'll find that a positive relationship with food and food preparation takes you away from plotting and planning that one free day of eating and leading you down the dark path of food fest thinking. You'll realize you can navigate through any occasion without diving into a vat of food and becoming comatose from food-induced fog, leaving you feeling shaky and guilty, and running to the next binge of sugar, salt, and fat.

You'll appreciate the connection between food and mood, knowing and understanding how foods work in a medicinal fashion.

And finally, the third section (*Turn the Corner*) teaches you how to embrace *heal from the inside out*, no matter where you are or who you are with and what's going on, by combining gratitude, God, and wholesome food. This will quiet the food fest frenzy obsession with cheat days, turning on peace and contentment by establishing a constant link to YOUR Supreme Reality. To do this, you will learn to connect to other people and to the sacred art of food preparation. By this means, you will be able to eat your way through any place, event, or situation—no matter what, or where you are—and NOT FEEL DEPRIVED. Self-care and self-love will move you away from shame, blame, and personal judgment as they relate to the cheat day mentality.

This section also explores grocery shopping and cooking to create the sacred art of mealtime—to learn that every day can be a good day as you eat your way through London, Wisconsin, Italy, or wherever your travels take you. Here, I wind down with some final thoughts on freeing you from making food your best friend, so that instead you can eat your way to inner peace and practice a mindful relationship with food

Often, while writing this, I have been asked by patients how this book ever came into being. I think the best answer is that after I wrote my first book, ***Release your Obsession with Food: Heal from the Inside Out***, I realized my work wasn't done but rather only beginning. To unravel and correct eating disorders takes tapping into the many realms of r*eleasing your* o*bsession with food to* r*eleasing* y*our obsession with diet* c*hatter*—which led to this third book, ***Release Your Obsession with Cheat DAZE***. I needed to help those in trouble with food to travel from eating disorders to eating recovery, from negative chatter to positive chatter, to unleashing the *cheat day* mentality by eating healthful foods no matter *where you are* or *who you are with*, whether on the weekend out to eat, or in another state or country, or even on a massive cruise ship plowing through the seas.

The latter, of course, is what blossomed into this third book—how to release your obsession with food on vacation, weekends, and holidays, birthdays—or any makeshift celebration you have conjured up in your belief system that hooks into a cheat day mentality.

You see, we become attached to ideas and never let them go, creating a reference system that turns into our way of thinking, behaving, and acting out. Just like Kinsey, who believed she couldn't be her authentic self if she didn't have the customary foods, allowing for a cheat day (week or month), when she went home to her country. She believed she wouldn't have the *experience* if she didn't dive into the food—making food the culture rather than the family and adventures she would most likely experience if she weren't in a food fog filled with guilt and self-disgust. Such a pattern could only cloud any opportunity to bathe in the love of family and connections with others.

That said, Kinsey suffered from binge-eating disorder with a long, long history of dieting and bingeing, followed by more dieting and more bingeing. On any given day, she might carry an additional sixty pounds, which was her "set-point" weight, the weight her body tended to align to. As she learned to break the negative pattern, she was able to move into a positive direction experiencing her family and culture with love, while eating the healthy versions of food, losing any and all self-degradation, replaced with self-acceptance.

Please note that eating disorders, mental illnesses, mood disorders, and addictions are serious and often require a village to conquer. You owe it to yourself to tap into a pool of help such as through psychotherapy, group therapy, sessions with a psychiatrist, and/or time spent in places of worship and with reference to your spiritual connection. Twelve-step meetings, books on the topic, and any other mode of help that fits your needs and preferences are definitely recommended.

Kinsey chose psychotherapy, hypnotherapy, and meditation along with any and all spiritual practices to work on her binge eating and addictive obsessions with sugar, flour, and wheat.

The end result I've tried to produce in ***Release Your Obsession with Cheat DAZE: Heal from the Inside Out*** is a blend of a spiritual slant on cheat day obsessions, together with practical, down-to-earth advice. I want to help readers learn how to live more fully day to day in order to break from negative, compulsive, cheat day mentality (or any form of free eating just for today attitude) no matter where they are, who they're with, or what weekend, day, country, state, or celebration is at hand.

Where to Begin…

To start the process of healing your thoughts and behaviors, begin with self-love and self-care. The essence of what frees the dieter is love. You can learn to love your body as it is now and move away from fad diets of cheat days into eating natural foods—to heal your body and heal your mind—*from the inside out.*

Americans are caught up in dieting and pursuing diets that make false promises. They can't stop chasing fad, quick-weight-loss diets, hoping that THIS TIME they'll break free from out-of-control thinking while body obsessing and longing for a cheat day fix.

And yet, at the same time, food is consuming their thoughts: when to eat, where to eat and how to get it, especially if it's a festive occasion or a made-up event that promises delights such as morsels of foods that will fill their sadness, lift their spirits, and bring unrealistic promises.

A conditioning from the past says that on a long weekend you're entitled to a cheat day. Or we're going to the movies, so come on—how can you have an authentic theater experience if you don't munch on buttery popcorn and a chocolate bar—just this once. That's part of the movie-house culture, and without it, you're missing the event.

The patients and people discussed in ***Release Your Obsession with Cheat DAZE*** range from individuals in their mid-teens to eighty years of age. All those mentioned in the book were acquaintances, people associated with twelve-step groups and/or those in psychotherapy. In accordance with twelve-step protocol and patient confidentiality, names have been changed and at times genders switched to keep each person, including acquaintances, anonymous.

Now, before moving on to Chapter 1, I want to give you an understanding of more of who I am and how I got to where I am today. Some parts of *My Story* are repeated from my first and second books, ***Release Your Obsession with Food: Heal from the Inside Out*** and ***Release Your Obsession with Diet Chatter: Heal from the Inside Out*** while other parts have been added with the goal of sharing another piece of me with you.

This is a book about getting out of your own way with food, weight, and fear in order to travel or spend quality time off without going into food-fest frenzy with the cheat day mentality. You can treat how you eat in the same way you would work your money to become debt free and financially comfortable. Calories and money run similar to one another in that spending money or burning calories cycle with acquiring money and calories. What you save with money provides opportunity going forward. What you invest with calories, or let's say quality foods, moves you toward better health, along with a release from your obsession about what and when to eat. Both money and health can bring you to quality living. If you take the step to change your foods, you move closer to a healthy lifestyle—the same with money—take the step to put away a little each week and watch what happens.

If you're looking for the roadmap to get you home, you've found it. If you're looking for something easy or fast, though, you have the wrong book. If you're looking for a book to help you become skinny in a nanosecond without effort, you have the wrong book. If you're looking for a medical guru to explain in depth the ins and outs of nutrition, you have the wrong book. But if you're looking for a book to lead you out of the cheat day, food fest frenzy no matter where you are, or who you're with, and you're working toward a healthy relationship with food, body, and lifestyle—a freedom beyond your wildest expectations, *long term*—this is the book for you.

I'm reminded of Dave Ramsey's, *The Total Money Makeover*, where he says, "This plan works, but it will cost you. It will teach you to say new words, like 'no.' In short, your Total Money Makeover will be a personal money makeover where you learn this motto: IF YOU LIVE LIKE NO ONE ELSE, LATER YOU CAN LIVE LIKE NO ONE ELSE." I say, "If you eat like no one else, later you can eat like no one else," meaning you will learn *your* personal roadmap that works for you with clean, whole, natural foods without pressing cheat day buttons. You may find this tough in the beginning, but once you work your program to your lifestyle, the freedom of living in a thin, strong, healthy body, no matter where you go, or who you are with, will be your reward.

I want you to know I understand all too well the hell of celebratory eating and cycling between the highs and lows of events all sprinkled with promises of love and happy dust if you eat this or that during this festive occasion. But luckily, I know the way out and wish to share it with you as I have with patients for the last twenty-three years.

Table of Contents

Part I

Cheat DAZE - The Food Fest Frenzy

Chapter 1

My Story

Touch the earth, love the earth,
and honor the earth,
her plains, her valleys, her hills, and her seas.
Rest your spirit in her solitary places.
~ Ernest Dimnet

Every food addict has a story, and I'm no different. Parts of **My Story** here are adapted from my first two books, as my story hasn't changed—though each book represents a different side of the diet mentality. My first book focused on the physical and chemical reaction to specific foods resulting in food addiction, while the second book looked at the "head talk" that dieters know so well. This book looks at any excuse to "party" with food, prompted by the cheat day mentality.

Food fests mean festivities or celebrations that lead to eating *because that's what we do.* In other words, time off from work or from an everyday norm can lead the foody into food fest frenzy with a cheat day plan. As we power through obsessions, our connections to family are more pronounced and transparent, unlocking our cultural associations and past festive activities.

Some of my fondest recollections of my childhood are of our family gathering together for mealtime. Sundays were often extra special when we might stop at Panozzo's for ciopa (pronounced with a sh sound—chowpa), which had a delicious crusty outside and white, soft bread on the inside. This bumpy/pointy-looking, flakey bread purchased on the South Side of Chicago in my Roseland neighborhood originated in the Veneto region of Italy. This went along with a stinky cheese (that's what we called it but I believe it was a block of sharp Parmesan cheese), a carton of eggs, milk, bacon, and Chicago Girls pastry—another favorite Sunday treat made up of a lovely flaky pastry. A brunch created for royalty. These are warm memories of an easier time before the neighborhood deteriorated, and we moved.

At such weekend events, the six kids in our family piled together at the table, waiting for a scrumptious breakfast. But don't let me fool you—we weren't a quiet bunch at home—only when out in public were we polished and presentable and well poised with the English manners my mother bestowed on us. During these Sunday festivities, my brother Michael would flick Danny, and Danny would kick Debbie, all while Mickey judged who was in the right and who was in the wrong. Christy was the eldest and didn't have time for child play—she grew up before her time. *I was the watcher.*

In a perfect world, mealtime is sacred time for family, conversation, and community. Some of my most cherished reminiscences are of our meals together, either on Stewart Avenue in Chicago or up at Grandma Baba's in Wautoma, Wisconsin. We sat down at her orange table speckled with colorful Fiesta plates, eating grapefruit, eggs, and blueberry pie—and burnt toast. Grandma Baba said burnt toast made your teeth white. Does it? I think it was her ploy to get us to eat the stuff. And the cute boy who came to deliver the milk with his father was icing on the cake.

Memories of meals flood in as I think of those days, treasured and confusing all at once. My Grandma Ruth could be volatile compared to her soft-natured mum, Baba—a "proper" English woman who emitted love just from her very presence. She had a soft but confident voice and held herself tall and well controlled. She was nothing but kind—a person of love, while Ma, my grandmother, not so much.

My grandmother, Ruth Stark Blodgett Risetter, was the person I most resembled in my issues with food and body obsessions, and sometimes in personality. The only difference is that I was fortunate enough to have "the awakening" and make profound changes in my life, whereas she didn't. Times were different then. The self-help, self-reflection, and spiritual boom hadn't yet taken hold. If it had, perhaps her story would have had a different outcome.

Grandma Ruth, who we addressed as Ma, was blessed with stunning beauty that well matched her muscular, toned physique from years of swimming professionally. She had the world by the tail. Ruth came from a well-to-do family of newspaper entrepreneurs and rubbed elbows with the town's elite.

Ruth's grandfather, Charles G. Stark, pioneer newspaper editor and founder in 1870 of *The Berlin Journal*—which came to be known as the "biggest little daily in the United States"—was loved by all, not only for his business sense but for his unshakable faith. He aligned with the Christian Science religion in 1903 and resisted catering to public opinion—whether regarding news, personal actions, or his belief system, all of which were intertwined. He was known around town as a "force for civic good and community."

Ruth, unlike her self-made grandfather who barely scraped past fifth grade, was well educated at the University of Wisconsin in the late 1920s, a time when women rarely attended college. She was beautiful, wealthy, and smart, and in love. She married Arnold Blodgett, her prince—a love short lived. Arnold, at forty, died of a massive heart attack, leaving behind his young wife and two teenage daughters.

Although Ruth appeared to have it all, her life had a dark side that became visible after the loss of her husband. Her relationship with food and at times alcohol was Ruth's downfall. Unlike those preceding her in her family lineage, Ruth was estranged from any spiritual underpinning. She wasn't a particularly kind woman, and her nasty, angry side magnified as she started to gain weight uncontrollably. When Ruth was in her forties, her body began to show the physical effects of carrying massive amounts of weight. With aching joints and a wobbly gait, often favoring one knee or the other, she was easily out of breath climbing up a short flight of stairs.

Ruth dieted constantly, only to regain any pounds lost, as she considered her next diet choice. From her late-thirties to her early-eighties, she maintained her miserable personality and went up and down in her weight—both behavior and pounds brought on by a chemical imbalance, her nemesis. Then, when Ruth moved into a nursing home run by the White Habit nuns who served only natural foods, love, and spiritual nourishment, she morphed into the sweetest, loveliest woman you could imagine, until the age of eighty-six, when she passed away.

It wasn't her fault…

My grandmother Ruth didn't particularly like me nor I her until her later years when I began to understand why she was an angry, bitter woman. The real tragedy is that if she had known what I know now, she (and my mother who showed a similar pattern of food abuse) could have been saved years of pain, out-of-control rage, and lifetimes of obesity. Early on in my childhood, I saw the glint in her pale-blue, watery eyes, a slight mischievous grin every time she talked about sweets and alcohol—a crazed-lust look—vicious and giddy rolled into one. She frightened me.

What I saw in Ruth, I saw in myself—a disconnect—unlike the personality of my great, great grandfather, Charles, who was always chatting and interested in anyone and everyone. He radiated true kindness. Love. He didn't seem to have the chemical imbalance my grandmother and I had. Unlike Charles, we were chemically, emotionally, and spiritually bankrupt. Perhaps you are, too.

My mom and Grandma Ruth were not so fortunate as to find relief; both died never to know the freedom of spiritual recovery, a quiet mind, or that their defeat in the battle to lose weight wasn't their fault.

By close to twenty-two years of age, my mother, Joan (Ruth's daughter), had given birth to six children. When Mom was seventeen, my sister Christy was born, followed by the twins Michael and Michelle eight months later. One year after that, Mom had another set of twins, Daniel and Debborah. And nineteen months later (with a miscarriage in between), I was born.

I was told that several of us were Southern Comfort babies, meaning that alcohol took over my mom's sense of worry about becoming pregnant. At any rate, as a newly converted Catholic, she didn't use birth control.

So, my mother was knee deep in diapers for what must have seemed like an eternity while she was only a kid. I learned early on to soothe myself with a bottle and food.

Although I was a scrawny child who was on iron drops for anemia, my dysfunctional eating behaviors were already developed. I remember climbing up on the kitchen counter to retrieve chocolate syrup and pouring it down my throat until I felt the sense of "ahhhhhhhhhhh" that food addicts are so familiar with. I was barely five. I hid in the dark hall closet and stole change from my parents' coat pockets to buy stashes of candy.

Once, I was so desperate I stole my father's pouch of parking lot change from the third drawer of the china cabinet—hundreds of dollars—and took it to Pennies to buy candy. I was seven and the bag was awkward and heavy to carry. When I dropped the bag, coins flew all over, and the storeowner turned me in to my parents. It was the first and only time my dad ever spanked me.

In third grade, I gave up candy for Lent only to sneak sweets during my 40 days and 40 nights of abstinence—certain God would punish me.

By the age of ten, I was adept at stealing money to purchase sugary foods, filled with guilt. Sneak eating caught up to me as I turned thirteen when my hormones raged out of control. My body began to grow, and I found myself a full-breasted woman with a little kid tucked inside of her.

My Diet Days Begin

I learned early on that bodies were a topic of open discussion from others. That bodies were critiqued and measured by a certain look and shape—and that faces were scrutinized too. That beauty was more important than the inner soul of that person—though my awakening later on taught me otherwise. Some people, such as my grandmother and mother, never get the awakening.

My grandfather, Nono, on my dad's side, was from Caldogno, a province of Vicenza in the Veneto region of Northern Italy, today with a population of 11,291. Nono was a handsome, dashing, suave, girl-magnet kinda guy. He loved women, family, and food, all part of his Italian heritage.

My sister Debbie and I spent many weekends at Nono's home, my Nona Anna Maria already having passed on August 28th, 1946—ten years before I was born. Both Debbie and I habitually stretched out on the big cushy chairs watching television favorites such as *Tarzan*, *Casper the Ghost*, and *Lassie* (a Rough Collie) with his companion Timmy in one adventure after another. Those were easy times—simple times, and food was never an issue.

Nono had an open kitchen, granting us the opportunity to eat anything and everything to our hearts' delight. My all-time favorite was vanilla wafer cookies dunked in Ovaltine with a raw egg cracked into it. I know…I know…it does sound gross today, but at the time it was considered a treat—and so *good for us*. As Nono would say as he urged us to indulge, "Mangia, mangia!" Ovaltine is still promoted as a health benefit for children and adults alike. I recall the chocolate malt-like taste that brought instant comfort.

Unlike the adults at home or any other place I can call to mind, Nono loved children and loved to see them eat. He had an open refrigerator policy, and we took advantage of that. He was warm and kind with an overabundance of love that came with hugs and a hearty laugh.

Shortly after the time of those tender memories, my siblings and I were whisked to our summer cottage to live, leaving behind my grandpa, who then moved into a nursing home facility due to Parkinson's, and our lovely neighborhood—where everyone came and went from one home to another as doors were never locked—shifted to an unsafe place and time. The year was 1969—a tumultuous time in our country.

Being in Wisconsin and living at the summer cottage year-round was quite a transformation from the comfortable life we knew in Chicago. At twelve years old, I seemed to grow up overnight—leaving behind toys and familiarity, and most of all childhood—a simpler time.

The memory of riding in my brother Michael's freshly painted, bright-orange, 1950s milk truck, as he took us siblings to and from Wautoma High School is a fond yet scary recollection for me. He drove fast and furious in a vehicle that could easily tip over.

Back in the day, a milkman would deliver milk and other eatables to people in their homes. The truck was designed without doors in the front so the milkman could quickly slip in and out from one delivery to the next. The engine was powerful and loud, causing the entire vehicle to vibrate.

We sat on the humps above the tires, holding onto the makeshift handle hanging over us for dear life while bracing our legs firmly on the floor, swaying back and forth with every turn, stop, and twist the truck made. Although I should have been petrified, I was mostly thinking about what I could eat NOW and how fat I was getting.

My inner prattle was mine: mine alone. Nobody was aware of my ongoing distress—my negative brain chatter—the tug of war between whether to eat or not to eat. I NEEDED sugar, salt, and fat, and yet I HAD to get thin. Food meant fat.

Nobody knew of the chaos in my mind—they had no idea I suffered in confusion with my thoughts. I lived in two worlds, one in which I acted as if I were present, nodding to indicate I was taking in what was being said or what was going on around me, while the other, highly agitated self existed in an inner-mind struggle far, far away from the here and now.

That memory of riding in my brother's truck is of my inner jabbering consumed with diets, with the intention to get thin yet planning for my next cheat. I obsessed day and night about how "fat" I was and how skinny I *needed* to become. Yet I was nodding and laughing with my siblings, who also were hanging on for dear life, fearing this massive milk truck would tip over any moment.

My negative diet obsession began when I was thirteen years old. I believed I was disgustingly fat and would only get fatter.

I weighed 115 pounds.

This insane thought process became inescapable. It was the start of my binge eating and excessive dieting followed by cheat days that turned into a gorge and my becoming numb and dazed. I ruminated I MUST BE THIN…no matter what. Well…the more I thought about it, the bigger I got. I was hanging onto something that was manifesting in a direction the complete opposite of what I wanted. I was so fearful of getting fat, that's exactly what happened.

I ate my way to two hundred thirty-four pounds, and for years went up and down in weight. I never remained at my highest weight long, but the stay was long enough to torture my soul, until one day, in my early thirties, I began to catch a glimpse of what I needed to do. But then I took still another ten years to completely let go of my diet mentality and crazy negative inner mind chatter to release the internal noise and move into freedom from this devil grip.

My craziest diet at seventeen was nothing but Ritz crackers and cream cheese, hot tea with skim milk, and Sweet'N Low. I dropped fifty pounds in six weeks—and began to lose my hair in patches, along with my short-term memory. My face took on the texture and color of a pasty, soggy cracker while my eyes sunk inward—framed by dark circles. My moods vacillated from deliriously happy to utterly miserable. Then, when I broke down from food deprivation and resumed eating, the pounds returned—*and then some.*

I went on to diet pills and any wacky diet I could find. In this way, I gained and lost fifty to a hundred pounds at a time for years—losing weight temporarily and regaining more than was lost. Each diet failure left me a little more bruised mentally and emotionally: and larger physically. I felt worthless and fat.

Fortunately, in my late teenage years, I found my way to Weight Watchers and began to lose weight and build confidence, and my mood swings were less volatile. The original Weight Watchers' program back in the mid-1970s, under the guidance of Jean Nidetch, the founder of the organization, followed a "natural" food path adopted from diets used for diabetics in a hospital setting. *I instantly felt relief.* Little did I know back then that I was sensitive to "processed" foods, which led to binge eating and crazy inner dialogue.

I reached my "healthy" goal weight for the first time at the age of nineteen, and I stayed there and basked in my glory for a whole five minutes. I then gained most of the pounds back after reintroducing sugary foods following the maintenance program. I went on to reach my goal weight three more times, and in my thirties, I finally was able to maintain a hundred-pound loss for ten years by following each new and improved Weight Watchers' diet—armed with willpower and a clenched jaw.

With my false sense of success, I went to work for Weight Watchers, thinking I had finally found my solution. But once the novelty of shedding weight had lost its punch, periodic binges, mood swings, terrible fatigue, low self-worth, and low-grade depression again resurfaced, not to mention that the negative inner diet chatter went from a whisper to a roar.

Through diet and exercise, I managed to keep my weight down but not without a terrific battle with binge eating and a string of typical food-addict head games. For several weeks, I ate according to the Weight Watchers' food plan (which after the 1970s Diabetic Hospital Plan introduced boxed desserts and pasta delights!), then binged on large amounts of sweets and starches over short periods of time while telling myself I deserved to eat—promising to begin my diet the following day.

Out-of-control eating gradually allowed my weight to creep back on, a pound here and a pound there. Before I knew it, thirty-five pounds had found their way back, and none of my old promises to myself worked. I was petrified that I was headed for a return to daily binges and on my way up to two hundred thirty-five pounds. Even worse, I was in graduate school studying to become a clinical psychotherapist with a focus on eating disorders and mental illness. I was the expert, yet I drowned myself in food. I sought education and information and used a blind trial-and-error approach, while I strove to find answers for individuals who had the same issues I had.

Eventually, I became conscious of a change in my behavior and moods with certain foods, as well as constant fatigue with specific foods. Some foods were so powerful they compelled me to eat enormous amounts, leaving me high, while others simply knocked me out. In either case, I lacked control. These foods induced anger, anxiety, low self-esteem, and negative inner diet chatter that was controlling, not to mention terrifying. This discovery was a tremendous breakthrough. My predicament wasn't my fault. I wasn't weak. I had a definite reaction to certain foods.

Still working for Weight Watchers while studying for my Master's degree in mental health, I noticed I wasn't the only one going up and down the rollercoaster of how I ate—so were many Weight Watchers' members as well as the staff. I knew they were trying to "diet" the weight off, and like me, were running through the revolving door of Weight Watchers to find the resolution to a weight-loss impasse.

I knew intuitively the answer wasn't just in following the plan, because as wonderful as the program was (and still is), it didn't provide an educated, licensed psychotherapist. A psychotherapist could have walked the members through the *why* they were eating, as well as *what* they were eating, though most wouldn't actually understand the situation if the member had a food sensitivity.

I knew I had to do something about this terrible problem for both myself and for others, so with great trepidation, I left the fold that had initially showed me the way. I was frightened!

I felt as if I were leaving the mother's womb as I stumbled off into the dark alone. I took with me little guidance, except knowing that certain foods were causing me to react with extreme highs and lows, and that my spirituality, which I had been brought up to respect, was stagnant because I couldn't see past the next binge.

With awareness, I developed a list of the foods that profoundly increased my cravings, mood swings, and a serious case of fatigue. After I'd worked with hundreds of patients and weight-loss participants and attended a regular twelve-step meeting to fill my spiritual deficit, I found unambiguous answers, and knew I was on the right path at last. I learned, too, that I wasn't alone. The inner chatter was beginning to quiet.

I isolated three specific ingredients that gave me the most egregious side effects: sugar, flour, and wheat. I found when I ate a balanced breakfast, lunch, dinner, and snack, and avoided sugar, flour, and wheat, while at the same time moving toward my Spiritual Source, my moods stabilized, my weight dropped, and I stopped bingeing. My cravings disappeared, my energy soared, and my depression lifted. And the inner noise began to quiet from a shout to a whisper, to barely audible.

My weight and my relationship with food were a constant struggle for me until I began to understand my chemical reaction to certain foods. After years of trial and error, research, clinical knowledge, weight loss, and stability of weight, I became calm. These days, I follow a simple formula, breaking down each meal in terms of structure and commitment rather than eating randomly. I also include daily exercise such as walking or biking along the ocean, and try and live my life as a prayer.

No, I am certainly not perfect (and realize I sound as if this is so easy), and my life isn't always bliss. I would love to eat any food I want, but I understand the consequences aren't worth the indulgence. I do feel angry when I'm tired and work too many hours, or when I have to turn down an invitation to an event because the atmosphere won't be conducive to my food needs (and bringing my own foods is inappropriate), or when everyone will be eating a delectable piece of chocolate cake and I take a pass.

But no matter what struggles life presents, I know that binge eating simply is no longer an option for me. Nor are sugars, flour, or wheat on my food list, because I understand that the sleeping giant within (addiction) will wake, and chaos will return with a vengeance if I ingest any of these. I compare my situation to that of a heroin addict who can't have just a smidgeon of heroin; he must abstain completely to stay clean.

When I began to follow these specific guidelines—even when I didn't want to—my negative mind chatter quieted, and for the first time in many years, I could become still and hear the infinite spirit's whispers. I connected to my inner strengths, and a pure understanding emerged in me. I found internal peace, transcendence, and love. Love for myself, others, and the universe evolved inside me.

Not only was I calmer, kinder, and less self-centered, but I began to see a bigger picture. I saw food as real and not real: nature's food and man's food. I chose food of the earth, sea, and air rather than processed and boxed. I turned to my Mystical Source so that the "noise" in my head ceased, and the addiction flattened. These days, I eat to live rather than live to eat. Healthful foods and a refreshed belief are now my fuel to optimal health and weight.

Make Way for a New Path

As quoted at the start of this book, "Do not go where the path may lead, go instead where there is no path and leave a trail."—Ralph Waldo Emerson. Let's make way for a new path now. Create a new way of looking at holidays and weekends and long stretches of time, without making it all about food. The phrase, do not go where the path may lead, in the context of this book is saying to break free from what you always do.

Let's break free from what always was and create a new path for what will be. A new path frees us of all the burdens of giddy obsessions about what gooey foods to eat because it's vacation time. Clear the path.

Emerson's wise words are a key to halting our inner mind war to open a new self-dialogue and invite success into every fragment of our being. This recipe of clearing the path of old to create the path of new is of paramount importance. In this way, we may gain access to a fresh way of handling the wide open space of time off with a transformed "vacation mentality." We can begin to look at food as nutritious as well as delicious, no matter what else is going on.

Imagine what you would feel like if you didn't fall into the diet on and diet off mentality just because you have a long weekend ahead. Instead, you can make the weekend about time off to be with loved ones, or read a book, or explore your town's events—without diving into a vat of food and numbing out with a sugar-laden treat just because you have free time.

Our goal is to move out of cheat day mentality and to look at our getaways with a revised lens. The outing is not about food but about the awareness of where you are and who you are with. Real self-awareness lies in connecting to the here and now. When we numb with foods that we think ARE THE EVENT, we miss the moment. Can we live in the moment if we are numb, in a coma state as we meander through the vacation?

Ideas for connecting to your real self and your surroundings are sprinkled throughout these pages; a dusting accompanies each word with the hope of liberating you from all the weight and pain of life you have suffered, as you release your obsession with cheat day behavior once and for all. You no longer have to be the food fest prisoner longing for the upcoming cheat day. You know, the one festering for foods that you ***think*** you must have because everyone else is having it—or because you deserve it—or heck because you're on vacation—or because you scheduled it.

My discussion to come portrays two adjacent worlds—one stuck in the "gotta eat this stuff because otherwise I'm missing out," the way Kinsey felt, obsessed with compulsive negative behavior—and the distinct world present in the conscious mind of quiet inner calm, connected with nature and the spiritual self—and with other humans (and well-loved pets). You owe yourself the opportunity to stay in the here and now and embrace the moment, not the food.

Most often, nobody knows about the insane, chaotic chatter in another individual's mind—they have no idea the tormented person is in two worlds, the one in which she is *pretending* to be present and the other in which she is knee deep in an inner struggle, far, far away from the current reality. The goal for us is to step onto the conscious plank of the *now*—not yesterday or tomorrow, or the fabricated story running amuck in the mind.

Over and over again, patients tell me about the money they're going to save, the weight they're going to lose, the book they're going to write, or the business plan they want to ignite. But in many instances, the plans and dreams keep being interrupted or dismissed because they are waiting for the *right conditions.*

When is it the right time? When is it the right condition?

Don't fret that the conditions have to be perfect. No such thing as perfect may ever appear. The truth is, you are *still* going to have to take that first step. If you take it now instead of later, you will be that many steps closer to your ability to handle any festivity by making healthy food choices this time next year.

Congratulations, you've just taken the first step investing in yourself by purchasing this book! You are well on your way…

My hope is that what I've written helps you to recognize, deal with, and resolve obsessive vacation/eating mentality—and transition to living in a more spiritually oriented realm. If my journey lifts and releases you from the pure hell of destructive food fest frenzy, I will, indeed, have accomplished my goal.

Now is the time to dial down the obsessive food fest frenzy each time you have a celebration or a break from the normal work week. In Chapter 2, we take a peek into Cheat Day mentality, which is most likely the underlying connection to the vacation food frenzy mentality.

Personal Inventory Questions

1. We all have a story, so what's yours? You picked up this book because something resonated within you. Are you a food fester?—meaning every celebration no matter how big, no matter how small is an invitation for you to cheat.
2. In what ways are your eating patterns similar to those shown in the chapter? When did you first notice you couldn't stop after just one cookie or potato chip, or whatever your addictive food was/is?
3. Often we have a family member we don't much care for—they rub us the wrong way. Upon closer look, what ails us about them may be what we don't like about ourselves. They mirror something about ourselves we don't like, or perhaps *we* mirror a distasteful part of them. What family member do you most resemble? How do you feel about that person?
4. Events and festivities often mark or define our relationship with food, confusing the actual situation with the *feel good*

feeling of certain foods. Can you recall a favorite childhood family food event? Who was there? What made it special?

5. Do you find you have foods you're sensitive to? What foods are they, and what happens when you eat them?
6. Do you have a history of your weight fluctuating up and down? When did this start? And did festivities bring this to your attention?
7. Do certain foods make you feel terrific—no cravings or mood swings, just a stable centered presence?
8. Do you have a history of food issues in your family? What about eating disorders or addictions of other sorts? Where do you fit in?
9. When was the last time you created a lovely meal and shared it with people you loved? Was food guilt involved? Did you experience shame, blame, and self-judging? Did you mix your own disdain for yourself with the event?
10. Reading a book such as this can teach you how to handle issues around food and move you beyond where you've ever been in your history with foods and celebrations. Imagine no more white knuckling your way through an event, and what a peaceful, confident person you could be. As you prepare to read through *Release Your Obsession with Cheat DAZE,* what do you hope to accomplish? Can you picture yourself enjoying those times of food challenges without even thinking about food?

Chapter 2

Cheat Days

We are all inventors,
Each sailing out on a voyage of discovery,
Guided each by a private chart,
Of which there is no duplicate.
The world is all gates,
All opportunities.
~Ralph Waldo Emerson

It was the end of my workweek, and I had one patient left to see: Sally. Sally, a lovely freckled-faced woman, of Irish descent, full of life and fervor, bounced into my office, seemingly delighted it was Friday. She had a giddy smirk, a glint in the eye, as she settled into the couch, pushing back her seat in a recline position as if to say, *Hey, it's the weekend. Let the party begin.*

You see, Sally followed a strict eating regimen, that was, until Friday night, when she'd meet up with her boyfriend as well as a small group of friends at various restaurants and eat whatever she pleased. And this Friday was no different. She was chomping at the bit, impatient and eager to get to her dinner, avoiding eye contact with me, or even discussing the plan when I gently brought it to her attention.

Sally knew I'm not a fan of cheat days. And she also knew every Friday she falls into the same trap of cheat day mentality. She plans for the one day to eat what she wants. Cheat day is an expectation of eating out-of-the-norm, highly processed foods, *on purpose,* with intention, in a conscious state of mind, for one day out of the seven. The idea is to quarantine one day for allowing any and every food of desire to be eaten as Sally so chooses.

Why am I not on board with a "free" day of eating whatever you want? Because, this thought process turns into something other than the intended outcome. It becomes breakfast, lunch, and dinner, snacking throughout the day on high calorie foods—all the foods you think you might have missed out on during the week. The mentality that ensues is about "catching up." People under the influence of this type of thinking go from cheat day to cheat days to cheat DAZE—a complete zombie state after consuming toxic foods.

Most important, a food sensitive person, binge eater, or any type of eating disordered person is NOT a candidate for a "cheat-day" program. *Not ever.* Why? Because this group of people, me included, is chemically charged to react to any sugary, floury, wheat-type of food—and with the cheat day mentality of grab and gobble anything, these are the "go to" foods, for sure.

What do I mean by chemically charged? Experiments with animals and humans show that, for some people, the same reward and pleasure centers of the brain triggered by addictive drugs like cocaine and heroin are also activated by food, especially highly palatable foods such as sugar, fat, and salt. (More discussion on that in Chapter 11.) Like any addictive drug, these very appetizing foods trigger feel-good brain chemicals such as dopamine.

Kathleen DesMaisons, PhD, in *Potatoes Not Prozac,* notes that because of what and when they eat, a sugar-sensitive person's blood sugar can't be counted on to remain stable and give them a reliable and steady source of energy. And Kay Sheppard in her *From the First Bite: A Complete Guide to Recovery from Food Addiction* states that the biochemistry of food addiction follows a path, which starts when refined carbohydrates flood the brain with dopamine, serotonin, and norepinephrine—all neurotransmitters (chemicals found in the brain). Up and down you'll go, from highs to extreme lows as if you were on a teeter totter. Though the food ultimately affects your mind, the problem is not a mind issue but rather a food issue affecting your mind.

Cheat Days Turn to Cheat DAZE

Sally's cheat days originally started with her intention to eat free on Sundays. She ate whatever she wanted and then promptly returned on Mondays to eating her scheduled foods. This worked fine *in the beginning*, though against my advice.

Sally has a long history of binge-eating disorder—eating large amounts of food in a short period of time several times a day, week after week, month after month to the tune of gaining hundreds of pounds. Desperation filtered in, and she turned to weight-loss surgery, for which she was an excellent candidate. For the most part, she then worked a healthy eating regimen, leaving her only twenty pounds from her ideal weight.

All good you say? Well, no, not so good, because Sally has food sensitivity, or to put it bluntly—she is a food addict. When Sally eats sugar, flour, wheat, or any type of processed foods, she falls off the *clean eating cliff* and enters the *anything goes* agenda. Not good. And when she caught the cheat-day wave, her weight began to climb a pound here and a pound there, putting her at risk of returning to her all-time-high weight nearing 400 pounds on her five-foot-six frame.

So, here comes Friday, and there goes Sally with her cheat-day mindset, "*But it's only tonight,*" she says with a clenched jaw.

"But tonight is Friday, Sally, and your 'cheat day' is isolated to Sunday only, right?" Sally waves her hand into the air as if to brush me off as she continues with her happy banter and not-so-happy recounting of the week.

So it goes…cheat night turns into cheat weekend for weeks on end until the weight inches up high enough to terrify Sally, and then she reins it in and begins to eat healthy but while extremely restricting food. Hmmm, sounds like diet mentality to me. I could see the morphing of a trend to a cycle of on and off—diet and not diet, to restricting—coming into fruition.

In Chapter 5 I discuss diet mentality. Diet mentality is a tough one to get away from. It's so tough that I wrote an entire book about it: *Release Your Obsession with Diet Chatter: Heal from the Inside Out.* Diets don't work. They fail, and the eating frenzy once again soars its ugly rage. And for certain, cheat days don't work. They turn into cheat daze—it's a setup for disaster—in time.

Cheat days are the flip side to diet days. It's a ping-pong game—back and forth and forth to back again. The cheat day mentality doesn't result in any change in behavior for the positive because the reward for "being so good" is to have an entire day to cheat and eat what you want. Oh yeah, it sounds great but the reality is that with it comes the guilt and shame as the dance of good and bad and right and wrong begins. Cheat days and weekends…sounds a bit like food fest frenzy to me.

We are all inventors, each sailing out on a voyage of discovery, every one of us guided by a private chart of which no duplicate exists. The world is all gates, all opportunities, as Ralph Waldo Emerson pens.

Sally has her personal voyage of discovery guided by ***her*** claimed compass. Her journey is to discover the world is all gates—all opportunities. She will make mistakes and corrections. She will learn the waters and discover that an all-inclusive healthy lifestyle will provide a freedom she never knew existed.

The Lie

The lie is that you will be able to eat the nectars of cookies, cakes, candy, ice cream, and chips *this one day,* and then you'll be able to go on and eat your well-orchestrated foods. But the missing link is that those rich, processed foods open the valve and the flood rushes in…the seas become rough and non-navigable and Sally begins to experience this sinking, drowning sensation that steered her to the gate of weight-loss surgery not so long ago. Her surgery, too, was the promise of opportunity but only if she restricted her foods to minimal amounts of calories, making her feel punished in that she couldn't eat like other people.

Cheat days are not the promise they make themselves out to be.

I once was lured into the magical thinking the cheat day mentality brings. The idea I could eat anything and everything for one day was glorious. It blared the trumpet of a freedom, a promise that sounded like a slice of heaven. To imagine I could eat what I wanted for one day, returning to my healthy eating on the remaining six days and continue to lose weight or maintain weight, depending on the case, was a food fest dream come true. Sign me up!

My weight began to creep up a pound here and a pound there to the point of 34 pounds *above* my one-hundred-pound weight loss almost a half a lifetime ago. I was exercising to the tune of three hours a day, but that weight kept inching up. I couldn't understand this. The promise was if I ate healthy six days and exercised moderately—and surely I was not, as I over-exercised—I *would* lose weight.

The Promise of P. K. Smith

What changed? Why was I gaining weight all of a sudden when I'd kept it off for quite some time with only bouts of overeating here and there? Now, all of a sudden, I returned to bulimia through exercise and eating out of control more often than not. My downfall all began while listening to the promises of a certain talk show host, whom we'll call P. K. Smith. In my thirties I was hooked on his message and his assurances. His promise was: *You can't fail. We've made a diet breakthrough, a cutting edge above the rest.* He was good. And to date, he still touts the same old message. This is not to say his plan isn't good for some because it surely is—just not for the eating addicted person, food addict, eating disordered, including those who are beset by bulimia and binge eating and excessive exercising, as a bulimic-anorexic individual will be.

I listened faithfully to the weight loss guru I'd heard on the A.M. radio station when I was driving to one of the weight-loss classes I taught back in the 1990s. How ironic—I'm teaching weight loss for Weight Watchers of Greater Miami, listening to Mr. Weight Lifter. He was on every Saturday, and I made sure to tune in. He promised that if you ate protein and veggies—no starchy carbohydrates but rice and never fats or fruits or bread of any kind except on Sunday, your cheat day, that you'd be able to have the life you wanted.

I wanted that life…

What he described sounded like pure heaven, a food addict's dream come true. Think of it, it'd be like telling hard-core alcoholics they could have their whiskey every Sunday—as much as they wanted—and then return to no alcohol Monday thru Saturday. Oh yes, please, I'm in!

One Saturday I worked up the courage to call the 1-800 number advertised and made an appointment to meet with this guy. After meandering through twisting and winding roads in a warehouse development, I stumbled upon the place. There, P. K. Smith greeted me with a firm grip, warm smile, and crisp blue eyes, standing about an inch shorter than I. He was bulked, sporting his gym clothes attire. His office was filled with weight-loss products such as weight-loss balls, pulleys, assorted machines, protein shakes and powders, and several of his books.

My takeaway that day was eat whatever you want on Sunday, and you'll lose the 34 pounds as long as you eat on a restricted plan during the six remaining days, exercise, and never waver. I questioned him about people with eating disorders, as that was my field of expertise, and he dismissed me, saying that wasn't his area. So, big book tucked under my arm, I left with a vision of sugary, starchy foods dancing in my head for each and every Sunday.

The idea sounded like a dream come true. For once I could live like a normal person and enjoy foods others ate without going off the rails. His idea of eating freely one day a week and staying on point the remaining six made great sense to me.

Once upon a time I smoked cigarettes. I know the habit wasn't smart, but it was cool back then, and I thought smoking would keep me from overeating. No. But before the realization dawned on me that cigarettes wouldn't keep me thin, I was hooked. I chain-smoked until the age of 29, when I got quite sick after drinking rusty water. The bad water caused an intestinal poisoning, and the idea popped into my head that the time was optimal for quitting the nasty, expensive, cancer-causing addiction.

I soon hurt in every part of my body, not only from the intestinal poisoning, but also due to the withdrawal from the nicotine. When the craving for a puff would stir, I'd think, *If only I could have just one a day*—just one. One cigarette a day is sort of like one potato chip—can't eat just one. And similarly, the cheat day concept runs to being doomed to failure.

Then with my new diet plan from this radio weight-loss guru, when Sunday came, eating whatever I wanted seemed ideal, but I ate like an eating-disordered person on a binge, chowing down on every delectable, sugary, fat-laden, salty food I could get my hands on; and then with clenched jaw, I went through six grueling days of eating the plain, sandpaper-like foods I'd assigned myself. Sunday couldn't come fast enough. And when it did come again, I went to town, eating this, that, and everything in between.

The Brick Wall

Like Sally, I soon after that hit the brick wall. My Sunday became Saturday night *and* Sunday and then it became *Friday night and Saturday and all of Sunday*, and with this revised, unwise program came the shame, guilt, and out-of-control eating. And of course the weight gain.

Though Sally didn't sign up for the P. K. Smith rally, or even know about handsome P. K. and his promises, she grasped this concept through the internet as she surfed the net one lonely Saturday afternoon. She read, wide-eyed and hopeful that she could have her cake and eat it too—so to speak.

Sally banked on her weight-loss surgery to "fix" the issue, but she learned fast enough that this wasn't going to be the situation. She needed to incorporate lovely, well-balanced meals, in her case due to bariatric surgery, four to five times a day every day for all the days of her life, along with moderate exercise and drinking plenty of water. A cheat day was not in the cards, as it would lead to out-of-control eating, surgery or not.

Weight-loss surgery makes eating larger volumes of food more difficult so the day's menu is broken into smaller meals, which is more digestible. The dietary intake comes down to a simple number-balance game, without processed foods, including sugar, flour, and wheat. Once Sally was finally on board, she was fine. She learned this soon enough, so that the cheat days became a thing of the past.

Weight-loss surgery can be a lovely tool to start the patient on clean eating, plus adding in a healthy lifestyle, including moderate exercise, a spiritual practice, and real food. All is well when this style of eating is the everyday practice, whether the day is Friday, Sunday, a holiday, or a day on a cruise. But somehow, the lure of *I can eat anything because I've had the surgery* takes hold, and down the murky waters the patient goes every time. Soon old habits resurface and excess weight is restored.

And cheat days may work for some, but I assure you if you're in the categories mentioned earlier such as someone with any eating disorder/food addiction, you, too, will disappear down the rabbit hole. Thinking you can win at cheating just once in a while is like expecting to win at the slot machine if you feed it twenty dollars and pull the handle. Chances are really good you will lose those twenty bucks and then some. A free ride simply doesn't exist, but a healthy way of eating delightful foods can fuel your body, sustain your health, and open the valve to healing on the inside as well as the outside. Now this is a promise that's true time and time again.

The world is all gates, all opportunities, as Ralph Waldo Emerson puts it, so what are you waiting for—taste life rather than yearning for processed foods, and just wait and see what gems lie ahead you.

The goal of this entire book is to help you break free from the food fest frenzy that cheat days, whether for one day or for one occasion such as holidays, weekends, or travel time and getting away to the getaway discussed ahead in Chapter 3.

Personal Inventory Questions

1. Do you think cheat days have any validity? Have you ever tried to eat whatever you wanted for one day, then return to your regular, regimented eating?
2. We are all inventors, each sailing out on a voyage of discovery, guided each by a private chart, of which there is no duplicate. What voyage of discovery are you on?
3. The world is all gates, all opportunities, as Ralph Waldo Emerson pens. What opportunity awaits you?
4. What part of Sally's story hits home for you? Do you become giddy at the idea that you can eat freely for one day?
5. The internet is an information highway at your fingertips twenty-four hours a day, seven days a week. It never sleeps. What cheat day idea/concept did you stumble upon there? How did you steer away from it? If it pulled you in, what did you learn about yourself?
6. Radio, isn't as impactful as the internet but is a close companion as it also touts promises every day, at all hours. What commercial might have pulled you in? How is it working for you?
7. And yes, we have the television with its one million channels beckoning with promises of solutions. Which one called you and how did its claim resemble a cheat day?
8. Do you believe the food fest frenzy starts with the idea of eating whatever you want but for only one day? What part of that calls to you?
9. P. K. Smith has been in the weight-loss/body perfect business as long as I have, and he's successful. What part of his message do you find dangerous for you?

10. Rather than a cheat day, what would it be like for you to every day create lovely meals that you enjoy yet don't crave or come to fall into the rabbit hole after you partake?

Chapter 3

A Getaway to Get Away

Live in each season as it passes;
breathe the air, drink the drink,
taste the fruit, and resign yourself
to the influence of the earth.
~Henry David Thoreau

In *Release your Obsession with Diet Chatter: Heal from the Inside Out,* I wrote a chapter on "A Getaway to Get Away," of which I've included snippets here, as the chapter prompted this book, *Cheat Daze*, concerning food fest frenzy mentality. Just because you're experiencing a long weekend or an outing or celebration of some sort, don't think you're given a free pass to enter into a food coma for days on end. Instead, practicing the art of getting away can be a healthy spiritual exercise. As Thoreau says, *Live in each season as it passes; breathe the air, drink the drink, taste the fruit, and resign yourself to the influence of the earth.*

Years back, when I worked for Weight Watchers of Greater Miami, I gave a talk on celebrations and eating. I started with January 1 New Year's Day, and went on to February 14

Valentine's Day, to March or April Easter/Passover celebrations, to Memorial Day weekend and Labor Day weekend, with the 4th of July sandwiched in between. On the board I created, I made room for birthdays, Presidents Day, Martin Luther King Jr. Day, Christmas, weddings, funerals, summer vacations, and winter break, along with spring break. Soon, barely a week peeked through the markup without an event of some sort, all of which most likely involves food.

The lesson here was, those who are seeking a reason to eat what they shouldn't will always hit on a getaway or celebration that lends itself to cheat day mentality. When I was writing *Release Your Obsession with Diet Chatter: Heal from the Inside Out*, I realized my work wasn't done with diet chatter alone because along with an obsessive focus on "dieting," "events" draw the would-be cheaters away from healthy eating,

Since that chapter morphed into this book, I have included my thoughts here, in *Releasing Your Obsession with Cheat DAZE*, as well. And oddly enough a real-life, ground-level storm (a hurricane) is brewing now as I write, one year later, as it was back on Memorial Day weekend when I wrote the original chapter. Yes, that's right—I live in Florida.

A Snippet from *Release Your Obsession with Diet Chatter*

Off in the distance, across the water, multiple conversations linger in the air as different households party down on this Memorial Day weekend 2018. I can't make out exactly what they're saying since competing music drowns out their words, but the laughter and occasional shouts of joy are clear. Though I'm alone this holiday, my heart is full as I take in the joy from their parties filtering through the breeze. I love to sit out during a warm evening on my three-person, cushioned canopy swing, swaying under the twinkling stars, but tonight, ominous black clouds cover the sky.

Tropical Storm Alberto is predicted, yet nobody seems to care or be paying attention. The festivities continue, and the small boats power by, all oblivious to the almost Category 1 hurricane forecasted.

Interestingly, I started the book *Release Your Obsession with Diet Chatter* during Hurricane Irma, which whizzed through on my birthday, September 9th, 2017. We live in an evacuation zone, forcing us to stay farther inland. Our son Benjamin and his wife, Zoe, graciously opened their home to me and my husband, Joe; older son, Kris; Oliver, my Eclectus parrot; and Southern Grace, a bouncy Swiss white shepherd puppy. Though the power was out a good portion of the time during our stay, we managed to busy ourselves.

Each of us meandered to separate corners to read, scroll through our phones, and eat, until eventually the storm lulled everyone to sleep. So while all were drifting off into sweet oblivion, I began *Release Your Obsession with Diet Chatter: Heal from the Inside Out.*

And here I was during another calendar event (Memorial Day), once again pounding the keys with another storm looming.

Boom, Boom, Boom go the competing drumbeats and clinking of glasses accompanied by hilarity ringing out across the waters. Despite all denial, Alberto is soon to pass through.

In between raindrops, the celebration continues.

Getaways are good. Good for the soul. As Rumi says, "Don't sit and wait. Get out there, feel life. Touch the sun and immerse in the sea."

Live in the moment, as life waits for no one.

Getaways don't mean you have to physically get away. You can get away exactly where you are. But breaking away from our everyday world and breathing is essential. We must step off the merry-go-round of life and tap into awareness and gratitude.

To stop the inner chatter, we sometimes need to move away from the norm. We need to become aware of our surroundings…breathe…love…and look after our anxiety. Embrace our pain.

While my fingers pass over the keyboard, I wonder about the story behind all those people across the way as their laughter rings out. Are they really happy, or are they intoxicated? How do we get away from the norm without numbing ourselves with drugs, alcohol, and deep-fried nibbles?

How to Get Away

Sit, listen, dive in, and watch the healthy escape begin. Breathe it in…you don't have to do or say or be anything in particular. Just step away from the everyday norm and live in the moment. Yesterday is gone; tomorrow has not yet arrived—all you have is now. Just be. It's good for the soul.

Although I write this piece at my getaway place, getting away isn't necessary in order to enjoy a getaway. Wherever you are, whatever you're doing, you can get away exactly at that moment in that place.

How, you might ask. How can I get away when I have dishes in the sink, laundry to be washed and folded, bills to pay, kids screaming in the background? Simple. Put on your walking shoes and escape through your front door into nature's natural getaway. The trip is free, and it's yours, no matter where you are or what else is going on. Leave your phone behind. Unplug from devices and plug into the earth.

Take a long walk with no destination—no end intended. Just walk. And allow your thoughts to roam, exploring what you see. Let your mind rest. Let your chatter still. Look at the flowers…really look. See the colors. Get close and smell God's perfume. Feel the breeze against your skin. Hear and watch the birds as they sail overhead. Feel the warm sun against your skin. Feel your feet moving over the pavement. You don't have to go anywhere special. You don't have to be anyplace in particular. Just be. Feel life in the now. Okay, so you say you can't walk because of your bum knee or sore back or other physical concerns. Not a problem. Get away exactly where you are right this minute.

Just sit and breathe. That's really what meditation is all about. You don't have to buy expensive how-to videos on meditation. Simply sit and let go. Take in a long, slow, deep breath, eyes closed, and see where the journey takes you. You don't have to think about anything or anyone just to breathe. Soon, you'll experience whatever you're supposed to experience. Meditation isn't forced or controlled or completed in a certain way. Do it your way—without worrying about right or wrong. Just sail off on your journey into the mind.

So maybe you're thinking, yeah, but what about the mind chatter going on inside me? My mind chatter won't stop, and you want me to meditate!

Yes, practice sitting in a quiet space for a few minutes at first, and then build on that start. In time, you'll work up to ten minutes, then fifteen, and so on. When you begin thinking about your bills or tasks you have to accomplish, remind yourself all those details will be waiting for you to handle later on, but it's not for now. Push back your daily concerns by going to your happy place.

Happy place? you ask. Yes, we all have a happy place, even if we have to make it up. Maybe you read a great article about a spot you've always wanted to visit. Make that your happy place. Feel it, embrace it, smell it...own it. The mind will switch to happy from a mere single happy thought. Studies show when we think of a puppy or a kitten, instantly a brain shift occurs. You will go from melancholy to happy, or from angry to content. Something fires in the brain. It's love. Love fires in the brain, simply by thinking about *your happy*, whether real or pretend.

My happy place is right here at my beach house on the swing or on the dock, looking out over the water. Whether I'm physically here, or just here in my mind, I switch on the happy button. Many of my childhood memories, good and bad, were, and are, tied to this very space I sit in while writing this section. I love it here. The setting is on the water, with family and neighbors living more outside than inside. Unlike when we're in our primary homes, where most of us don't even venture out, here at my getaway, we all live life outside in nature more than inside.

I'm never alone here, even when I'm alone. Inevitably, the homes across from mine and adjacent to it are lit and filled with activities, whether on a holiday weekend or not. The attraction that pulls us together is the water where dolphins shimmy by, seagulls fly overhead, and boats weave in and out of the Gulf of Mexico.

Sitting now on the swing, I hear the parties continue on. Though I'm not a part of the hoopla, still, I feel connected. It's my happy place and I don't have to do anything while here. I pull up on a Friday, never to get into my car again until Monday, when I head back home.

But when I'm back to my weekday life and need to quiet the chatter, I take in a few long, deep breaths in a comfortable chair, or wherever I am, and think of the dock or swing, and voila I am there: my family breach house. I can arrive in one second flat. *Let the meditation begin.*

Meditation on the Go

Okay, so you say you're not too sure about meditation, that sitting still in a quiet space without your mind churning is hard. Well, then start with something known as movement meditation: Meditating while moving.

Walking, as described above, is my favorite form of meditation. Other types of movement meditation practice may include walking through the woods, gardening, qigong, and other gentle forms of motion. I have one patient who absolutely switches into a meditative state when she's home alone cleaning her house from top to bottom while listening to hard rock as high as the volume can go. Okay…that would NOT be my happy place—but we all have our own view of happy, and this is her way of magically transforming her irritable state of mind to blissful joy.

Movement meditation is good for those of you who find peace in action rather than in sitting still, and for those of you who prefer to let your minds wander.

You can also take a yoga class for your getaway. Yoga is a form of moving meditation. While doing your yoga, you may feel parts of your body move in ways you never thought it could. Now stretch and reach to another level beyond your comfort zone. Escape the now as you know it, and experience your body. Connect to your body. Your size or your age or how flexible you are don't matter. What matters is connecting to yourself and escaping the inner noise.

My first experience with yoga was on the eve of my birthday many years before, when Zoe, my son's then girlfriend and now wife, bought me an "action" present. She loves giving "action" gifts, something that we can do together rather than an individual gift. I wasn't too enthusiastic about this particular present as I tend to be clumsy and thought I wouldn't get this yoga stuff, and most likely would topple over in sheer embarrassment. Nonetheless, off we went to yoga with my new yoga mat and yoga clothes. We were to do this under the stars at the edge of the beach, with the Atlantic Ocean in full view. And this particular night was the night of a supermoon.

A supermoon is a full moon that coincides with the moon's closest approach to earth. On the night of this supermoon, the moon appeared larger and brighter than at any other time—and I was told a supermoon is surprisingly rare.

The larger-than-life moon was so bright it lit the whole beach. This was a magical start to my first yoga experience, barefoot with the still-warm sand beneath my mat. I had the calmest, most unusual emotion I'd ever had. Yes, I did topple over—and more than once—but it didn't take away the most amazing feeling I'd ever experienced. I was connected to both my body and the earth simultaneously. It was pure heaven.

Okay, so maybe movement meditation or going to a getaway place isn't optimal for you. Consider prayer.

Prayer

Prayer is a powerful getaway that can be undertaken no matter where you are or who's with you or whatever else the situation at hand may present. Prayer is free. Prayer can come in many forms, in many ways. Prayer can be a conversation with God or your Higher Source of understanding. Think of it as talking to your closest, dearest friend who holds no judgment. Prayer is a spiritual communication between you and a source greater than you.

There is no right or wrong way to pray, but rather prayer can take any form that feels comfortable for you. You can use a prayer from childhood or a prayer you learned during your twelve-step experiences. Or you can simply talk to your Higher Source. Knowing you are not alone, that you can hang out with your *confidant*, provides an excellent getaway that you can make a part of your everyday, minute-to-minute, life. Prayer is not meant to be complicated; it's merely a way to open the door to your Source.

Living life as a prayer is certain to quiet the screaming voice in the head.

So maybe prayer is foreign to you or not something you're comfortable practicing, but for sure you don't have to travel to a place of some sort to arrive at your getaway. You don't have to go to Hawaii, or Australia, or lovely Italy to find your peace and quiet....though all of those places would be divine. Your vacation can be a staycation...exactly where you are.

No rules to getting away.

A Staycation

Make your hacienda your place of getaway by doing activities in your home or neighborhood, or checking out nearby attractions. Arts and crafts can be a form of a getaway. Or some people find escape in painting. I'm quite content painting a wall or a room or an old piece of furniture, and voila I'm in a getaway place in my mind, daydreaming about a whole lot of nothing—thinking how lovely letting the mind wander without worry or fear feels.

The other type of painting, the more artistic kind, will work as a getaway as well. Coloring and painting a picture are natural ways to move from the chatter in the mind to your childhood happy place. You can even color in an adult coloring book to escape from the mundane noises in your head. Studies show that the use of adult coloring books provide many health benefits.

Art therapy and adult coloring books are not quite the same as one another, though both are advantageous in connecting to our inner selves and moving away from the busy, noisy mind. But maybe the cost of attending art therapy or mingling with others in an art class isn't something that fits your budget—or your inclinations. And that's okay. You can tap into *your* version of art therapy using an adult coloring book. Some therapists have said that coloring has the potential to reduce anxiety, create focus, or bring about more mindfulness.

One of my fondest childhood memories is of a stormy day in Wautoma, Wisconsin, where we spent our summers. I was nearly eight only a few months before my beloved Baba (great-grandma) passed away. I loved her home, which was warm and welcoming.

Baba was the grandma we all would dream to have. She loved unconditionally. Many gatherings took place in her main dining room at the long, rectangle, burnt-orange table seating six children, Mom, Grandma Ruth, Grandpa Hale, and Great-Grandma Baba. We children often lingered at the table long after sharing a meal, taking in the adult conversation—family connecting, which seems so foreign today with fast food meals on every street corner to be eaten in the back seat of a car while Mom talks on the phone.

That day, we couldn't go out to play as the storms kept coming in from the west, and we were stuck entertaining ourselves. No coloring books were to be found, but my sister Debbie and I discovered as long as we had Crayolas, we could entertain ourselves.

We sat for hours on end on the oval carpet weaved in soft gold-orange and red earth tones with our warmed red faces hovering close to the fireplace, dripping crayon wax on two empty Coke bottles. Soon, engulfed in the sweet smell of melted crayon, burnt logs, and the fresh rain scent lingering from the outdoors, we forgot we couldn't run out to play.

To date, I have those very two bottles on my dresser to remind me of one of the happiest days of my life. The world felt right. We made a getaway right there on the floor, dripping and mixing one exotic color after another, while Cuddles, our cocker/spitz, inched close to the warm fire to dry her wet coat. I can still smell the melted Crayola and wet fur, while off in the distance the smells of dinner swirled in the air.

But maybe coloring is not your way to get away. Then sing…

Change the Channel

Sing…sing…sing. Sing happy songs and watch your getaway begin.

Maybe you have trouble quieting the old movies in your mind. Sometimes, scene after scene of what an ex-boyfriend or a love said to you, or of a sibling who stole from you, or of a parent who couldn't love you the way you needed to be loved will play over and over in your mind. And the pain is intense.

Perhaps your movie is saying, *If only I had done things differently* then my life would be better, richer, happier… Really? Maybe it would be worse. You don't know. It simply never spun out the way you wanted it to, whether reality based or not. So, how do we quiet the *what ifs*, *should ofs*, and *could ofs*? Change the channel on the movie in your mind. Switch to another thought.

Did you know you can't have two different thoughts at the same time? If you're singing your happy songs, you can't have a sad-melody mind monkey making music simultaneously. If you *think* about the mountains and you're sitting at the edge of the cliff swinging your legs over the edge, taking in the lovely earth below, you're sure to tap into your happy self. You are *there*—even if you're sitting in your car in the thick of traffic.

A getaway is from wherever you are in your mind. The getting away lies in redirecting your thoughts. A physical getaway may be optimal, but *in your mind* takes you there too.

Think positive, you become positive. Feel, taste, hear, and smell your happy place— and you are there in a nanosecond.

Don't let the past create your future. If you're conscious of this behavior, you can stop. You're allowed to make another choice. You can forgive the past and embrace the *now*.

Take note that anger, resentment, fear, jealousy, envy, worry, doubt, mistrusting are all emotions that can feel very real to you at the time you're experiencing them. But truth be told, they're of the mind, giving you reason to hang on to yesterday or live in tomorrow.

I'm not saying don't feel your feelings, because you surely should, but please don't let them own and define you. Take a moment to feel the emotion and then move through it to the other side where the sun is shining, the flowers are blooming, and the birds are singing. The time has come to get away to your getaway.

Again, at the risk of sounding repetitious, you don't have to go away to get away, I assure you. You can get away exactly where you sit right now while reading these words. Try it.

Close your eyes. Take in a deep breath. Find your happy place. Think about that place. And soon you will feel as if you're there.

Breathe in joy.

Smile Your Way to Happy

Why not smile? Yep, just stop what you're doing and smile. Do you feel the lift? Smiling has the ability to stimulate the endorphins in our brains. You don't have to think about anything, just smile, and the change simply happens.

Smiling can trick your brain into happiness. Science has shown that the mere act of smiling reduces cortisol levels. When we smile, our brains release neuropeptides, a nerve protein that influences our brains, bodies, and behavior in many ways. Particularly, this negates stress and elevates our moods.

If that weren't enough, when we flash happy smiles across our faces, we release "feel good" neurotransmitters, including dopamine, endorphins, and serotonin. The neurotransmitter dopamine gives the brain energy and motivation—a rush that is necessary for a habit change. At the same time, endorphins lessen our perception of pain, triggering a positive, euphoric feeling in the body very much the way morphine does. And serotonin, a confidence booster, seeps into our very essence, changing our overall moods.

Give it your best and make it a toothy smile. We take life too seriously.

Richard Carlson writes in *Don't Sweat the Small Stuff…and It's All Small Stuff*, "One of my favorite posters says: *Life is a test. It is only a test. Had this been a real life you would have been instructed where to go and what to do.*" He goes on to say, "Whenever I think of this humorous bit of wisdom, it reminds me to not take my life so seriously."

My sister Mickey has the most infectious laugh I've ever heard. She loves to laugh. She laughs freely. She laughs often. And she laughs loud. I'm more subdued and quiet, but not when I'm with Mickey. I start laughing. Laughter is a great getaway from reality, from taking life so seriously.

Have you ever watched a young child having a laughing fit? He falls to the ground because he feels the laughter in the core of his being.

When was the last time you laughed? I mean really laughed. Laughter is one of the quickest ways to dull the inner chatter and escape to another place—a quick getaway right in your mind.

Laughter is powerful and healing. Smiling is contagious. Try smiling at everyone you see today and I promise if they're looking at you, they'll smile back.

When I went to Italy with my sister Mickey; her husband, Emil; their daughter, Jacqueline; Jacqueline's husband, Trevor; and their three children: Vanessa, Caleb, and Colton, we all laughed. Everything turned into a funny. We were living in the now and embracing whatever came our way. Yes it was a getaway getaway, where you get on the plane and go somewhere foreign, but the real getaway wasn't that part of it…though that was amazing…but the laughing we did was what made the trip so spectacular.

Silly things made us laugh, such as my sister, who doesn't speak a lick of Italian, first introducing herself to our relatives we'd never met before as Michelina. Michelina!! Who the heck was Michelina? Later, we learned that was her Italian name in school at St. Anthony's when we were little bitty kids.

Anyway, Mickey was talking to our second cousin Nikko, just reaching his nineties, and who doesn't speak a speck of English. They were nodding and bobbing their heads like a couple of pigeons and laughing to beat the band. What were they saying? Who knows? All I know is that later that evening we laughed and laughed, reminiscing, as we sat flabbergasted watching the two of them intertwining and connecting.

Lesson: You don't have to speak the same language to connect. And you don't have to be the same age or gender to bond. Laughter is universal. Smiles are universal. Kindness is universal. Where you go doesn't matter, either, or even if you stay right where you are. You can connect to people, animals, nature—your getaway is in experiencing the moment. Embracing the now is the ticket.

Hey, if you can get away to a real place that holds the key to your heart, by all means go. Each one of us can use time away from our familiar, everyday lives. But don't think traveling somewhere else is going to refresh you on its own.

I know plenty of people who go away on fancy trips, but they're still very lonely and caught in their "stinking thinking," as they say in the twelve-step rooms.

Calgon, Take Me Away

You'll find many getaways right there in your home. Yep, more escapes await you there in your abode. Your home *can* be an escape from the norm. Where? you might ask. Well, for one place, the tub—you know, that oval-shaped container with a flat base, found in most bathrooms.

When was the last time you soaked in a tub of hot water? The bathtub can provide a great getaway. Fill up the tub with hot water and sea salts with a few drops of your favorite scented oil, and you're on a fast track getaway from reality yet present in your body and mind.

It's no secret water has been used for healing, spiritual, and religious purposes traced as far back as the Bible. In fact, the Bible often references water as symbolizing faith and salvation. Throughout that good book, God uses water to explain His relationship with people. In essence, water not only sustains our bodies and communities, but also is an integral part of our spiritual lives. Water, earth's most abundant natural resource, not only covers about seventy percent of the planet's surface, it is a necessity for all living beings. Did you know the brain and heart are composed of more than seventy percent water?

So, a hot bath is a proper escape. A memorable vintage commercial back in the 1970s has never left my mind: *Calgon, take me away!* It so impressed upon me that hot baths could carry you away from all your troubles. Calgon Bath Beads, once thought of as a European luxury, became a household name.

Notice when you feel water against your skin whether in a shower, bath, or rain, or even after a jump in the pool, lake, river, or ocean, instantaneously, you feel better, lifted from the woes of life.

A Few Zs Anyone?

Another place in your home for a getaway is your bed. Yes, your bed can provide a getaway. Now I'm not talking sleeping for hours on end, which often comes with depression, but rather a nap. Nothing is more delicious than an afternoon spent reading an uplifting book, followed by a nap. If you watch your beloved dog or cat, they think nothing of taking naps. We don't have to simply sleep at night and then that's it.

Taking a nap is perfectly fine. A nap means sleeping for a short amount of time, thirty minutes to an hour. A power nap can leave you refreshed and alert, with improved mood to tackle whatever you have in front of you. It's an excellent escape—a way to hit the pause button—breathing newfound stamina into your day.

So you see, you can find many ways to get away to a getaway. I know you, too, know plenty of people who go away on fancy trips but, still caught in their cheat days mindset may wind up eating themselves silly. You might be one of them. Our goal is to remove the old thoughts and urges and replace that with calm.

And of course, some people get away to other cities, states, and countries and truly experience a quiet mind, just as I experienced a quiet mind coming to my beach house to my little getaway. I didn't need perfect weather. All I needed was some quiet time with a little laughter out in the distance as the parties continued. But soon I had to make my way back into inside as the rain began to fall, leaving behind the clinking of glasses and shouts of joy mingled with lively music as Alberto was kicking up the winds.

Let the storm begin.

Back inside, I was aware of the rain starting to pelt against the windows. The storm was coming, and being right there in my little getaway, exploring the quieting of my mind felt so right. Alone, yet never alone, always connected to the sounds of nature, whirling through its stormy self-knowing. Something bigger and grander than me is always present.

Getaways are crucial to a re-set from our everyday lives, and cruising the open waters (Chapter 4) is another way to do such thing without falling into the trap of cheat day mentality.

Personal Inventory Questions

1. Where is your ideal getaway place? What happens to you when you think about going there? If you don't have a place, then imagine one and experience it in your mind's eye. Where would you go? What do you feel like in this spot?
2. Getaways don't mean you have to physically get away. You can get away exactly where you are. But stepping out of everyday life and breathing is important. Why not step off the merry-go-round of life and tap into awareness and gratitude. Can you get away in your mind and tap into gratitude?
3. Can you imagine taking a long walk with no destination, no end in mind? Just walk. And allow your mind to roam, exploring what you see. What does that feel like to you?
4. As Thoreau says, "Live in each season as it passes; breathe the air, drink the drink, taste the fruit, and resign yourself to the influence of the earth." Live in each season as life pauses for no one. Can you live in the season? When was the last time you tried?
5. Take a yoga class for your getaway. Feel parts of your body move in ways you never thought it could. Stretch and reach to another level beyond your comfort zone. Escape the now as you know it and experience your body. Can you connect to your body? Does it give you an escape, a getaway?
6. What do you think about getting away in your mind simply by breathing and placing your mind on something other than the negative inner chatter? Sit, listen, and embrace it all to start. Breathe in, and no, you don't have to do or say or be anything in particular. Just get away and let whatever happens happen naturally. Letting go is good for the soul.
7. Did you ever think a hot bath could take you away from reality? Remember the commercial from years back,

"Calgon, take me away"? What commercial of the past really affected you? Why?

8. When was the last time you enjoyed a hearty laugh? How did it make you feel? Who were you with?
9. Do non-threatening storms give you some peace of mind? Do they quiet the inner chatter even for a moment? What is it about the rain that works or doesn't work for you?
10. If you could enjoy the perfect escape, where would it be to? Who would you want with you? Why?

Chapter 4

Cruising Open Waters

My soul is full of longing for the secret of the sea,
and the heart of the great ocean
sends a thrilling pulse through me.
~Henry Wadsworth Longfellow

The vast ocean spreading as far as the eye can see and beyond is magical and powerful, with stories and secrets extending back to the beginning of time. Longfellow nailed it. *My soul is full of longing for the secret of the sea, and the heart of the great ocean sends a thrilling pulse through me.* What makes the ocean so powerful—or so enticing? What, for many, is this call? Why does it send a thrilling pulse through most?

It's the water.

Human nature inspires us to turn to water for a sense of calm and clarity. People have known for millennia that being around water gives our brains and our senses a rest from overstimulation. Health gurus have said many times that staring at the ocean changes our brain wave frequency, placing us into mild meditative states. No wonder millions of people are attracted to cruises, and to boating.

Okay, so not only the water draws people to cruises—another attraction is the food. Yep, the food! The free-all-you-can-eat food. The idea that you can eat whatever you want, whenever you want lures people to the popular big vacation vessels.

I can't think of cruising without thinking of my daughter-in-law's parents, who are cruise-set kind of people. They know the ins and outs and all about(s) when it comes to cruising. Living in Florida, I observe that people here commonly choose to cruise for a trip. A cruise ship is a hotel on the sea. So the in-laws, who reside in the Central Florida area near the Kennedy Space Center, sometimes take advantage of this opportunity. Traveling to an accessible port to board is a less stressful option than flying off somewhere. Hence, because of the in-laws' love of big-time cruising, their daughter and our son learned to love the ships as well.

I've thus learned that cruise ships have all the amenities available for keeping up with a healthful lifestyle, including a wide array of natural and unprocessed foods, the option of requesting special menus (low-fat, vegan, what have you), a full-sized gym, aerobic classes, yoga, massage therapy, and swimming, not to mention a walking course, and on-land excursions like zip lining, kayaking, and swimming with the dolphins.

John, a patient who feared cruising as he had been in sobriety from alcoholism for five years, learned that he could find a twelve-step program on most cruises, while Chip, a known gambler in recovery, discovered meetings he could attend as well.

Though I live vicariously through others who are the cruise-set, I have my own boating stories to share. My experiences with vessels on the water are limited to boats where I spent summer after summer at Big Silver Lake, in Wautoma, Wisconsin since birth. Food, picnics, and boating all go hand in hand, whether the traveler selects a big cruise line—or a speed boat, kayak or pontoon—all promising the appeal of party-style food and drink.

I know boats as a passenger, as our norm was to spend endless hours at the lake skiing, fishing, and tooling around. As a driver of the vessel, or a passenger on the cruise ships, however, I'm a greenhorn.

On those long, hot, summer days, when I was a child, Mom would load the cooler with sandwiches, chips, and drinks for the day planned ahead. To date, I still enjoy boating, not as often, perhaps, but when I do I stock the cooler, too—but for me the contents are primarily fresh fruits, cold chicken breasts, Greek yogurt, raw veggie medley, and loads of water. Vigilance and planning go a long way toward having a health-promoting time.

Tide—What Tide?

Often "picnic food" conjures up ideas of chips and sandwiches, hotdogs and baked beans, topped with cakes and cookies, especially on Memorial Day weekend—the grand opening of summers. We imagine that without these foods we don't have a picnic, but of course this isn't true. You can have a delightful time on your outing eating fresh, real foods. Plan ahead, think real and not packaged, and you are well on your way.

My childhood friend and I decided to rent a boat on Memorial Day weekend though we had no personal experience piloting a boat, not to mention that we were toting along three very little children. We saw a cool island and thought to stop, eat, and let the kids check out the shoreline, stretch their legs, and collect seashells. We'd packed a lunch of fruits, fresh meats, and raw vegetables, along with gallons of freshly squeezed no-sugar lemonade, so this was as good a spot as any to set out our picnic supplies.

On this glorious day, we splashed, ran, and made castles and angels in the sand, with not a cloud in the sky, not a care in the world—*until* some burly looking fellas pointed, wide eyed, directly at our boat. Following their fingers, we let our mouths gape open as the boat was completely on the sand. How could that be? We, for sure, were responsible boat people. Ah, but we didn't think about the tide that goes up, and the tide that goes down.

Lucky for us, these strong men lifted our boat back to the water, and off we went, very relieved, until we realized everything looked and felt different at the low tide from the high tide. We had to call the Coast Guard Marine Rescue to come find us and escort us home. Good thing we'd fortified ourselves with delicious and nutritious foods to see us through.

Dolphins Dancing

Though I cherish memories of my mom and us kids boating together, our outings were never laced with real foods, but always packaged. Not uncommonly, boaters will stock up on beer, wine, crackers, and packaged/processed foods of all sorts. That these types of food are the foods to bring is ingrained in us by way of magazines, billboards, past history, etc. No. You can have wonderful times out with fresh foods, not missing those artificial, heart-clogging "treats" that promise nothing but headaches, stomachaches, or maybe even worse. Fail to plan then plan to fail…

I recall the time, when Benjamin was about eight, we took a rented boat to explore, and to our delight, a school of dolphins danced around our little vessel. The food we had brought included steak, apples, fresh asparagus, and homemade potato salad. Our outing was a real delight, as it reminded me of the many times I had gone on boats in this very spot with my mom before her passing, so we could observe dolphins. The excursion felt purely mystical when these special mammals circled the boat, as if to say: *We see you—and we know you're here, but you're safe.*

Memories of sad times or even good times don't have to be entangled in food to have important meaning. You can easily find clean, whole foods on a buffet. Look for real, stay away from sauces, sugar, flour, and wheat, and you are well on your way to a healthy outing.

But when the subject comes to cruising on big ships, the closest I ever came was the time my husband, Joe, and I joined another couple on a gambling cruise ship that sets out into deep, international waters for the evening. A band that my husband knew was playing drew his attention to the ship, so we went to support the event. I loved it!

The warm Florida breeze wasn't too cold and not too hot, and the lights sparkled, matching the glistening of the sea. The ship had a lovely buffet spread, and all the clean foods were easy to spot…alongside the processed foods. Try to do as I did that night: Glance over the foods, thinking balance, then create your plate with fruits, steamed and raw vegetables, baked or sweet potato, chicken, fish, or steak, and you're well on your way to enjoying the people and festivities with less emphasis on food.

Making the right choices was easy for us since our mindsets were fixed on clean eating as opposed to, *Let's cheat for one day since we're on this lovely boat—just this once.* Oh, the outing was good, until I turned and looked at my husband. All the blood had drained from his face. He was ash white. That was it—no more cruising in our forecast.

The Powerful Sea

When Joe, my husband, was young, he loved to swim in the sea with his friends on hot summer days during the times they weren't practicing music or playing in a club. They were teens who had started their musical careers early in life. On this particular day, however, Joe was stuck mowing the lawn as he'd promised his dad—though his friends were out swimming.

One of the boys never made his way back home. The tide was too strong, and he drowned. To this day, Joe recalls the sound of Mrs. W. wailing for her beloved son.

Since then, my husband hasn't been at all fond of the sea, water, or boats.

Emotions from the past often play into our current experiences, and such was at work that night he and I were on this gambling ship. Perhaps you have memories, too, that crowd your clear thinking when you go cruising or boating of some sort.

My soul is full of longing for the secret of the sea, and the heart of the great ocean sends a thrilling pulse through me (Henry Wadsworth Longfellow). The ocean is enticing and powerful, with a mind of its own.

The Dreaded Swimsuit

What about the dreaded swimsuit! Often, body image comes to mind at the thought of cruising or boating when donning the suit is part of the protocol. Perhaps you avoid the water at all costs due to your fear of exposing your body to possible onlookers. Making peace with our bodies is a first step to quieting the foodie within.

You see, food, body image, and weight tend to roll into one big challenge for many. But self-love and self-acceptance can be achieved, and you can quiet that negative self-reflection demon. Why not begin with a practice of appreciating your arms, toes, eyes, or hair to start the process of self-love. Give gratitude for the gift of a body with arms to hug, legs to hold you up, eyes to see, and a mouth to smile and laugh from. Move away from the desire for the body you *think* might be the acceptable shape that you need to be. Your body is your body for *you* to cherish, not for society to judge, or the magazine to decree, or anyone else to evaluate, for that matter.

Moving past your body image requires simple self-care, such as having a pedicure, brushing and flossing your teeth, and stretching and connecting to your body parts, appreciating each magical inhale and exhale.

Turn to the gift of being in the moment, in the now, rather than projecting a swimsuit fear that may or may not be based on reality. If it's real—you don't look "good" in such and such kind of suit—then find a suit that works for you. You'll be amazed at the different styles available these days designed for all types of bodies. And the suits are beautiful! Stand tall and feel good about who you are now—not tomorrow or yesterday or some imagined person who's not real.

Learning to navigate around this type of obstacle is the key to success. Yes, overcoming negative self-talk can be difficult when from our earliest memories we've been conditioned to think that we're flawed—not good enough. And the question is: by whose standards? Fuel your mind with positivity. Your health extends beyond your body, including your mental health; your physical health; and most importantly, your spiritual health.

Mara and Food Vigilance

And what about food choices on the cruise? Call ahead and make arrangements with the cruise line and even restaurants you intend to visit on land and ask what foods are on the menu. Remember if you fail to plan, plan to fail. Being armed with information and a strategy maintains the food as it should be and keeps the binge or "I don't care attitude" at bay. You already know the formula, simply plug that in wherever you go and whoever you're with, and you will succeed in eating nutritious, delicious foods.

Though I'm not Big-Cruise-Line savvy, I live by proxy through others who love to cruise, like my son's in-laws and plenty of patients I see. Take Mara, for example, my patient, who is a cruise queen, going to this island and that. Once upon a time, Mara thought of cruising as a food fest frenzy experience, a time for cheat daze. And her extra eighty pounds were proof of such thinking. She felt as I did in my first job at the local bakery—as though she had hit the jackpot—or was living a scene out of *Willy Wonka & the Chocolate Factory*. Food was everywhere Mara's eyes could see. She especially loved the chocolate buffet served nightly, laughing how she got her money's worth.

But soon the laughter ceased as she became heavier and heavier with each cruise experience. Mara thought of cruising as an invitation to eat. Her mindset was such that if the food is paid for, it should be eaten. This type of mentality is leaning on the edge of a great binge crash. Often buffet goers take part with the same attitude.

In fact, I was a buffet-driven girl, myself, at one time in my life. Every Friday for years on end I enjoyed "date night" with my sons, Benjamin and Kris. While their father was out playing music, we'd go to The Home Town Buffet, where we paid a set fee and ate until the cows came home. This went on for years until I had an awakening watching a good handful of significantly overweight, obese, and morbidly obese persons making several trips to the buffet, salivating over each treasure.

I *was* them, inhaling the sugary, floury, wheat foods as much as I could eat, way beyond full. The only difference was that my body frame was thin. When thin, you can go undiscovered. I was eating enormous amounts of food and later cycling for hours on end to burn through the calories.

My affair with the buffet ended on that last eye-opening occasion. Not to mention my older son bit into something inedible and fished out a red fingernail from his mouth. Done.

No more buffets for me on a regular basis. And for sure, no more eating my money's worth like Mara, because in the long run doing so is neither fun, nor healthy.

Together, Mara and I worked on changing Mara's relationship with and behavior around food. She began to own the concept that food isn't "bad"—it's a good thing and a necessity for life. Her perspective had been that if she ate "bad," she might as well keep on keep'n on, since she already had done the destructive thing. No, stop eating; regroup by evaluating and correcting—and then move forward.

Cruises don't have to be food fest frenzied but can be lovely experiences eating healthfully. You don't have to come back with the freshman fifteen, meaning that every time you go on a cruise you pick up fifteen pounds. Just as a student doesn't have to go to college and gain weight. The relationship with food, not the food, causes the hiccup. Plenty of enticing foods are healthy and good for you, as Mara soon learned.

To date, Mara cruises like nobody's business, but she eats healthfully. She looks forward to her breakfast of eggs, oatmeal with a dollop of butter, fruit, yogurt, and hot tea laced with skim milk—or a vegetable omelet with cheese and slices of melon. She knows now to pick from a list of morning foods etched in her mind and goes about her business. Lunch is no different. In fact, she feels like a queen, served with foods she doesn't have to cook or prepare herself, such as salad with chunks of chicken and avocado, along with tomatoes and slices of onion topped with olive oil and vinegar and a few pieces of blue cheese.

This method of eating works for Mara because she enjoys foods that nourish her and sustain her healthy lifestyle, no matter where she is—out on the sea, at home, or away for long weekends. She understands that the approach is about making choices and knows how to balance her meals.

Dinners on the high seas are always a delight of lobster or fish of some sort with browned garlic potatoes or sweet potato or even brown rice topped with sprigs of asparagus, or Brussels sprouts—or a large salad, with any of the other wide variety of colorful vegetables always at hand. Her half-meal is yogurt and fruit and she's totally satisfied.

Mara walks the ship every morning and sometimes joins the yoga group. She's convinced that when she's elderly, she'll be taking a permanent space in a room on the sea which she'll call home.

A cruise doesn't have to be a food fest frenzy but rather can be a getaway that's filled with peace and joy—fun and laughter—and good food that won't pack on ten or fifteen pounds or even two pounds, for that matter. It's business as usual wherever you are or who you are with. Again, once you clear the palate of processed fare, foods taste phenomenal in their natural state.

Is It Too Late for Love?

Chrissie was getting on in age, fearing her dream to see Europe was slipping off her bucket list as nobody wanted to travel with her due to their health issues. At the time, Chrissie was in her eighties, and with great sadness had lost her dearest travel buddies to illnesses and their passing on.

At one time, Chrissie held on to fifty extra pounds from all the traveling and eating she partook in, to the point at which she was suffering from high blood pressure, heart disease, and a serious case of asthma. She became very depressed, fearing her own health was declining, and that her life was virtually over, especially as she witnessed her friends becoming frail.

We began our therapy sessions with the goals of returning her joy and confidence in regard to traveling and living her best life, along with helping her knock off the extra weight she'd packed on from prior poor food choices. Chrissie loved restaurant outings, often choosing rich foods that she had trouble passing up or slowing down on regarding the amount eaten.

I conducted hypnosis sessions, offered confidence-building work, and helped her construct an eating plan that made sense to her. At eighty-four years young, she took the Mediterranean cruise she'd always dreamt of taking—though this one she took alone. It was the trip of a lifetime, fulfilling her bucket list with a stellar accomplishment—and finding love at the same time.

Chrissie met Bob, who also was actualizing his dream on the same cruise. Together, they bonded and have never parted since. Both in their early nineties now, they're cruising and partaking in all that life has to offer, believing you are never too young or too old to fulfill your dreams. Chrissie is fit, flexible, happy, and confident.

So if you are of the cruise-set or the just plain old boat-set, you can manage your foods, eating whole, clean, and natural foods in either case. Fail to plan, and you can plan to fail. Keep in mind, your foods are your foods—everything else is not. Take the same initiative Mara and Chrissie took, and you're headed for only good habits that will last a lifetime.

So, now that you are a master at making it in the open waters, how does diet mentality (Chapter 5) factor in?

Personal Inventory Questions

1. Longfellow nailed it: *My soul is full of longing for the secret of the sea, and the heart of the great ocean sends a thrilling pulse through me.* What makes the ocean so powerful—or so enticing? Do you share a love for the ocean? How does the atmosphere impact you?
2. It's been said that staring at the ocean changes our brain-wave frequency, placing us in a mild meditative state. Some even say just thinking about the ocean can change the brain

wave frequency, lulling us into that relaxed state. What are your thoughts?

3. To date, I still enjoy boating though not as often—but when I do, my cooler is stocked, too—but filled with fresh fruits, cold chicken breasts, Greek yogurt, raw veggie medley, and loads of water. Vigilance and planning go a long way. Do you plan ahead with food on your boating experiences?
4. Memories, good and bad can guide us one way or the other. My husband's experience with his childhood friend's unexpected drowning imprinted his mind, steering him far from the beach, boat, and cruises. Do you have a memory that catapults you into a good space, or bad?
5. When my youngest son, Benjamin, was about eight, we rented a boat—from the same place as with my childhood friend Julie. When we went out to explore, to our delight a school of dolphins danced around our boat, filling me with a magical feeling that makes me smile each time I think about it. I'm certain my brain waves are in overdrive as I visualize the dancing dolphins skimming across the water. What natural water experience comes to mind for you?
6. Have you mastered toting foods with you when on a boat outing? What fresh, real foods can you pack? Get creative, and you'll find a wide variety of foods that are delicious and fit your food plan while at the same time are inviting to your guests.
7. What about the dreaded swimsuit! Often body image comes into play at the thought of cruising or boating where donning the suit is part of the protocol. What is your relationship with your body and the swimsuit? What steps have you taken to connect with your body image in a positive way?
8. The buffet on cruise lines can be quite frightening for many. How can you plan ahead before ever making a food

choice at the buffet? Imagine the foods, as they are most likely the same wherever you go. Imagine your plate filled with clean foods, and that picture can become a reality for you.

9. What about Mara and her mastering of the cruise lines? At one time she saw the buffet and sit-down dinners as an excuse for a full-blown food frenzy, where now she makes conscious choices, ordering foods that work for her healthy lifestyle. What was your takeaway from any similar experience?
10. And can you find love out on the sea? Look at Chrissie, who wanted to cruise at 85…and boy, she sure did follow her heart, and fell in love at the same time. What's on your bucket list? Make it happen—it's never too late.

Chapter 5

Diet Mentality

Spring is nature's way of saying, "Let's party."
~Robin Williams

Spring, a time when the daffodils sprout, unfold, and blossom. A time when the birds start singing, and life is full of the promise of summer with picnics, long weekends, and vacations—all dazzling us. The message is it's "party time!" because that's what we do.

Spring is also the time when people jump on the diet wagon. Hey, it's summertime and you gotta look good in your swimsuit or swim shorts or whatever skimpy outfit people plan to wear. We can no longer hide behind the big coats, sweaters, and scarves. Our skin is bare, and arms and legs are exposed.

Look at any magazine at the checkout when you're at the grocery during springtime, or summertime, or even holiday times of any sort, and you'll see pictures of food and smiling, "thin" women on the front cover, insinuating it's time to eat—but don't worry because you'll be thin like the person in the picture *if you follow this specific diet.* ***Lose 40 pounds in three weeks!*** Yeah, right…I don't think so.

But then, look a bit closer, and see a headline promoting the diet that's positioned right next to the sweet-laden food, or the succulent loaves of bread, all dancing about the cover—and the woman with the infectious smile, with hands on her hips, leaning toward you as if to say, *"Do this and you'll be thin like me,"* as she flashes her toothy grin.

The message sent is a mixed one, for sure.

The message says it's summertime, and you need to put on your bikini when you attend the barbeque with hot dogs, baked beans, cookies, and cakes dancing about. Yep, you need to eat these things in order to have fun, ***but*** make sure you look thin and inviting too.

What is the message, exactly?

The message is that dieting brings happiness, and eating rich, processed foods brings happiness—a cheat day perhaps. Hmmm, how do we move between these two narrow lines, especially when vacation equals food and eating, yet we want to fit into the clothes that we chose just for the event at hand. Again, a mixed message.

Heck, look at the commercials featuring a hot, sexy girl next to the red, not-so-high-end car or even a high-end one, indicating if you buy this car you will attract a sexy girl. Sex sells. Fatty, gooey foods dancing on the front of the magazine, television, and billboards sells too, as the image screams, *Buy me and you will be this.* Whatever *this* is. Will you buy?

What about an average-looking girl carrying some extra weight, leaning against the non-impressive red car? Are the guys going to line up and buy the car? I think not. And what about the guy buying the car? Does he have to be a hunk? Nope, the *red car* will attract the girls, and a beautiful, drop-dead gorgeous, *hot* girl is leaning on the red car as proof of that. What a brain tease.

Diet mentality tells us: I'm going to get what I want in life if I'm skinny—but, simultaneously, I'm going to be happy if I eat this luscious treat—just this one more time. A vicious dance between how happy you are going to be if you eat this or that, but at the same time, you MUST be skinny if you are going to be happy. This is insane. You aren't going to be happy because you're skinny, or because you eat this or that. You may *temporarily* be happy, until the reality of life sets in—as does the hop from diet to diet, to binge after binge, with cheat days factored in.

What is the answer? The answer is to love yourself from where you are right at this moment. By now, you must be realizing here is the central theme throughout this book. Life and happiness are about now…not tomorrow, and not yesterday.

And how do you accomplish the now?

Coming into the now is all about self-care and self-love, right as you are. Yes, right now. You say, "But you don't get it. I'm *fat,*" as you grab a fold of skin from you waist. Ahh, but I do get it, as I, myself, once was you trying to "vacation" with all the dancing foods—and at the same time look skinny too. Yes, life lived in that manner was insanity, but your existence doesn't have to run that way. Yet the struggles come with the newest diets that keep popping up on the shelves, screaming you can be skinny if you eat in such and such a way.

And now, the newest kid on the block, is the ketogenic diet. Everyone seems to be talking about it—to the point that I hear a patient here and one there stating this diet is what he or she wants to try. I definitely respect every person wanting to try something other than what I prescribe. I do believe more than one answer is out there and finding the right prescription that works for you is essential.

And, YOU being the one to decide what works is imperative. I say, take what you need food-wise, self-love wise, and self-care wise, and sculpt it into the just-right formula for you. Then, you're in control, and you own what's going to work.

To Keto or Not to Keto?

The diet taking the world by storm and plastered all over the magazine racks, internet, and Amazon, as I mentioned above, is the keto diet, to some known as a ketogenic diet. Everyone who knows me knows I'm not a fan of fad diets—of any kind. They come and they go. But every now and then, one happens along that catches my eye. That's not to say I'm in on it, but I may be curious to see what the fuss is all about. And, the keto diet is one making a huge splash these days.

So, the question here is, to keto or not to keto? A few of my patients caught the keto wagon, so I decided the time had arrived to explore this new style of eating. I, at first, thought keto was the Atkins diet come again, since upon close look it seems to be—but it's not. Atkins promotes high protein, moderate fat and veggies, and low carb, whereas ketogenics seems to promote high fat, moderate protein and veggies, and no starchy carbs.

And then, in my quest to see what all the fuss was about, I stumbled upon *The Keto Diet*, which is an offshoot of ketogenics, or maybe the two intertwined. I have a bit of trouble saying exactly, as I see both discussed almost interchangeably. But *The Keto Diet* promotes unprocessed, high quality fats, moderate protein and veggies, and low carbs, whereas ketogenics is focused mostly on a high fat anything diet. Hmmm.

When these types of diet hypes pop up, I generally steer clear of even looking at them because they stir some old eating disorder stuff in me. As you know from reading thus far, I have a history of binge eating, food addiction, and bulimia through exercise, all of which I've been in recovery for over the last twenty-plus years.

One of the ways I was able to tame the binge giant was to eat a no sugar, flour, or wheat program, with a good amount of protein and veggies and moderate starchy carbs, fats, and fruits. And this way of eating has worked for me…and for thousands and thousands of people I know who struggled with addictive eating. I've seen so many miraculous changes in myself and in patients and in others I know, so that I've written books, such as this one, on the subject to share with the world.

Thus, to think maybe another way could be the answer piqued my interest. Could I be wrong, could another way work? In my research I looked into *The Keto Diet* by Leanne Vogel—and other diets populating the scene such as ketogenics—which seemed similar to me, as both promote high-fat eating. This category of diets touts the same good news that I scream from the top of the hill, but with a different food structure. How could this be? Could I be wrong? Are they wrong? Are we both right?

Perhaps we are both right?

This keto way of eating suggests it can lower irritability, stop the impulse to binge eat, promote weight loss, lower diabetic concerns, promote a healthy heart, and on and on, or so the promises go. Eating a balanced diet, such as I suggest, also lowers irritability, puts a stop to binge eating, promotes weight loss—but at a slow and steady pace—unlike the keto way, which appears to be fast and furious.

My concern with anything promising rapid results is that it may not be sustainable. Such an approach may be difficult to continue long term as a complete lifestyle change.

Removing sugar, flour, and wheat, as I suggest, also lowers diabetic concerns and promotes heart health, and much more—such as opening up a happy, freer you, connecting you to your higher self and Higher Source. Healthy eating—

moving away from the SAD (Standard American Diet)—is my mission for myself and for those I work with in a patient setting, from a speaker position, and through my books and blogs.

The red flag I have with ketogenics is the way it promotes fast weight loss and high fat consumption, with little room for carbs, such as fruits and starchy carbohydrates. *The Keto Diet* by Leanne Vogel seems better than most in that it promotes good eating from a nutritionist's view, with the focus on eating for nourishment and optimal health, though weight loss is a likely outcome. Leanne is authentic, open, and honest, admitting her flaws and mistakes with her version of the keto way.

But when Leanne promotes the fat bomb, consisting of avocado and coconut oil, or eating straight fat for an energy boost, my eyebrow does shoot up. Her sense of nutrition moves away from everything healthy I know. On one random podcast I listened to, she talked about how a girl ate a stick of butter and instantly felt better. What!!! Something about this doesn't sound good to me. And of course, with summer and vacations, and food all whirled into one, an idea like this gives me pause for concern.

As I've noted, *The Keto Diet* and ketogenic diets in general seem to be almost interchangeable. The keto plan seems to center on fat, which supplies as much as 90 percent of daily calories. Yikes!!!

Again, the promise of the keto way sounds similar to what I promote (stable moods, no bingeing, heart healthy, lowers blood sugar, clear thinking, etc.) sans the copious amount of fat, which is a frightening thought. I have this visual of bacon, butter, and cream, and loads of avocado.

My understanding of the idea of the ketogenic diet is for the dieters to drive themselves into ketosis, which occurs when your body uses fat instead of carbohydrates for energy. When the person is in the state of ketosis, fat eaten travels to the liver, which delivers byproducts called ketones; these enter your bloodstream, and are converted into energy. And dieters know they're in this ketosis state when their breath, skin, and urine produce an acidic odor.

I promote a healthy lifestyle through spiritual food, nutritious food, and moderate exercise—a body, mind, spiritual view. I'm not sure one can reach a balance missing any one of the three…sort of like trying to balance a four-legged stool on only three legs...wobbly at best.

We live in a fast-paced society, looking for quick and easy, and on some level, the keto diet seems to promise just that. But I'm not so sure. My instinctive feeling is that slow and steady wins the race. Anything worthwhile, and long-effect producing, requires time. Take writing a book: The process starts with that first sentence. If I hadn't written sentence one, way back when, producing my dissertation many moons ago, I'd not have three completed and published books ready to serve you.

Every journey, no matter how long the route may be, begins with that first step, that first word, *that first right food.* Begin with your first step, and you can build a new, authentic way of relating to your food as you vacation, celebrate an event, or join into upcoming festivities, without the cheat day mentality.

Practice self-love and self-care by eating nutritious, health-promoting foods, one bite at a time. Imagine soundness of body, mind, and spiritual connection. It's possible. But you *must* take that first health-promoting bite to begin your well-being journey. Once you do, each bite carries you closer and closer to your goal.

So is the answer to keto or is it not to keto? I think that's up to you. The patients engaged in ketogenics are losing weight—and fast. Working with me is not "my way or the highway"; the ideal path is for each of us to find their own way in this journey, making smart decisions. I don't know what these patients on the keto diet will look like or feel like down the road. Will they have a quick weight loss followed by an enormous weight gain? I sincerely hope not.

I gather from the hours and hours I've spent reading up on this way of eating and listening to podcasts, that those promoting this way of life admitted bouts of depression, weight gain, irritability, hunger, binge eating, and hair loss, along with other issues along the journey. So, perhaps the jury is still out.

Those I've known who have been eating balanced meals consisting of fruits, vegetables, protein, moderate amounts of dairy (if not sensitive), good sources of unprocessed starchy carbs, and fats, have grown into their right-sized bodies slowly and steadily—*and permanently.* Those eating based on *The Keto Diet,* as described in Leanne Vogel's books, seem to release weight steadily, and her focus seems to be on fostering a healthy lifestyle and being open to change—all good. So…there you have it…

I'm going with my raspberry pancakes made from oat bran, eggs, raspberry, cinnamon, and dark cocoa with a dollop of Greek yogurt. Oh yea, bring it on!

Raspberry Pancakes

Whisk two eggs, ½ cup of oat bran sprinkled with sea salt, cinnamon, dark unsweetened cocoa powder, and natural vanilla. Add one cup of raspberries and a teaspoon of unprocessed, organic coconut oil. Heat pan to the point at which a drip of water sizzles. Once the pan reaches the right temperature, divide into three round pancakes. Lower the heat, as it's hot enough now to brown. Turn the pancakes after a few minutes once browned and cook an additional few minutes. Enjoy topped with a dollop of plain, unsweetened, fat-free

Greek yogurt and sip a hot cup of tea—or decaffeinated coffee—laced with almond milk, and you have a perfectly balanced breakfast and content belly. Enjoy!

And Then There Was Lucas

Lucas, a handsome fellow who recently immigrated here from the eastern coast of South America sank down into the couch one afternoon, returning only weeks after weight loss surgery (the sleeve), grinning from ear to ear because thirty-five pounds had melted off his body.

The sleeve, also known as the gastric sleeve or sleeve gastrectomy, is a type of weight loss (bariatric) surgery that renders the stomach smaller—over half of the stomach is removed, leaving a thin, vertical sleeve, or tube, in place of the normally sized stomach.

Lucas finally had his solution to a twenty-year weight dilemma that appeared during his middle school years after he broke a leg on the slopes skiing, leaving him confined to bed for months, consoled only by salty, sugary, and fatty foods, bringing him to a catatonic state, hypnotized by the sugary foods and latest television series. He entered the cheat daze whirl.

When Lucas came to America on a student exchange program, he was introduced to the Golden Arches—a delight only the rich could afford in his country—and he ate and ate and ate to the point of piling on even more unwanted pounds. Try as he might, he could last on no diet for more than six months. Ah, but now he was riding the diet train, with built-in cheat days that would lead him to thin, once and for all, *because of the surgery.*

No. That's not how it works. No matter the surgery, you still need to let go of a diet mentality and grab on to lifestyle change. Erase the cheat day, and you erase the cheat daze.

Erase the diet mentality, and you birth the healthy lifestyle mentality.

I know you, yes YOU, the reader, are saying, but of course diets work, and without cutting your intake of food, you'll only gain the weight back. Okay, sort of, but understanding food intake in a prescribed way that becomes automatic is the answer.

Ouch, that sounds harsh doesn't it? What I just said sounds as though the answer lies in restricting in a robotic kind of way, but that's not what I mean by a "prescribed" way. The prescription is more like a formula that you ascribe to on a daily basis, that *naturally* becomes your norm.

Diets die. And a cheat day leads to binge eating. This sweet Lucas was now eating one thousand calories a day, primarily protein. He had been told carbs are bad. Fruit is a carb, therefore bad. Sweet potatoes are carbs. Bad. He was already in trouble before beginning. He needed a wide variety of foods, and the idea of taking off cheat days propelling his motivation to diet was a recipe for disaster.

Whatever you do to lose weight is the way you keep it off. I'll repeat that: ***Whatever* you do to lose the weight is the way you keep it off.** Think of Kinsley, introduced earlier in the book, staying on a restricted diet of only protein shakes and bars in Panama while her family was digging into rice and beans and savory chicken topped with all the decadent childhood treats she remembered. Give her two days, and she'll most likely cave.

Kinsey feels not having a cheat day isn't natural, and Lucas says eating like a *normal person* isn't natural. Hmmm, what about, *eating restricted isn't natural.* My South American patient won't survive long-term on a diet mentality of one thousand calories a day. He needs to cast his food choices wide, eating fruits, vegetables, protein, good sources of fat and starchy carbs, along with dairy—and then it is doable, palatable, and most importantly a "travel worthy" plan…

You're going to travel, have long weekends, celebrate birthdays and deaths, climb mountains and swim in rivers during holiday breaks, and eating just a tad of food won't cut it—not for the long haul.

Put away the diet and take out the food—real food—and learn how to combine and mix and satisfy your needs. Avoid becoming hungry by eating sensible meals throughout the day, and you're well on your way, no matter where you are or who you are with.

I Deserve a Cheat Day

What do you eat when you're enjoying a long weekend and you've worked hard and want to sleep in and then go out to breakfast? And you have the "I deserve something yummy" attitude. Yes, you do, and I do too, but not with a cheating attitude—a "just for today" way of viewing what you eat. So let's go to the drawing board and look at food and food groups.

A simple formula is to eat three balanced meals and one half-meal that some call a snack. But watch the word "snack" because it's a trigger for popcorn, chips, pretzels, and such, and that's not quite what your half-meal should be. The goal is to always feed the brain the right foods so you don't *jones* for other foods, and cave.

So let's begin with a simple breakdown of foods, and then we'll move into the lovely breakfast when you go out, based on the foods your prescription suggests.

A healthful breakfast consists of a piece of fruit—an apple, half-melon, bowl of cherries, blueberries, etc. And alongside the fruit, you might want protein such as eggs, tofu, leftover steak, or some other type of protein that's palatable to you. Then a starch, like rolled oats, corn grits, potato, or sweet potato with some sort of fat. Perhaps your fat is coconut oil or butter or maybe a slice of avocado. And top it off with a dairy of yogurt or slice of hard cheddar or mozzarella—you get the idea.

Now, visualize those foods in a way that's frankly delicious: an omelet stuffed with avocado and cheese and maybe sliced apples and chunks of sweet potato drizzled with olive oil, and voila you've made yourself a perfect breakfast.

Let's peek at lunch—another simple formula you can mold into a delectable meal: protein, vegetables, and fat. Simple. A stir-fry, consisting of: asparagus, mushrooms, onions, and shrimp, or any other combination of protein, plus a good source of fat and veggies. Use your imagination. Keep it simple. Keep it appetizing. Keep it real. Keep it as your arsenal to take with you wherever you go, and whoever you're with.

Your half-meal can be eaten in the late afternoon, or late evening, depending on what time you have your dinner. I'm a late eater so my half-meal, or "metabolic boost," as I like to call it, comes at around five o'clock in the evening. Notice I said "around." The goal is to space your meals *about* four to five hours apart to avoid the dip in blood sugar, and to avoid becoming ravenous and throwing out the idea of healthy foods, eating whatever is in front of you, regardless of what it is.

Okay back to the half-meal. You could take a cup of plain, fat-free yogurt, mix in a cup of blueberries, a tad of real vanilla, and perhaps a teaspoon of dry instant coffee and a tad of sweetener…mix and place in the freezer, to be eaten and savored as a frozen delight.

The dinner formula consists of protein, vegetables, starch, and fat. Simple, right? That's the goal, keep it simple, and then set your creative juices flowing. A dinner could look like: salmon, mixed spring salad with loads of raw veggies to your liking, brown rice, and olive oil, or whatever fat you find tasty.

So that's your set of formulas. Now let's get back to you rolling out of bed Sunday morning after a late night out, and you want to go to breakfast with your friends. Perfect. The time is late morning, and you make your way to your favorite restaurant, Joe's Café. You're starving.

Your first inclination is to scan the menu. Don't! Instead, scan your head and figure your foods out from your allotment. What does that mean, you might ask? Well, you know the prescription, so why do you have to scan the menu to confuse yourself? You know you're going to have protein and fat and fruit in the morning, vegetables in the afternoon or evening. Break that list apart in your head.

Just about every restaurant has eggs, chicken, fish, steak, hamburger, salads, olive oil, blue cheese, tomatoes, potatoes, (both sweet and white), along with fruits. So just start building from what you know. You can formulate a lovely meal that fits your eating style without feeling deprived or left out. Ordering a meal takes practice, perseverance, and a knowing of how to move the foods around. And sometimes you might be combining a breakfast or a lunch (brunch)—or a lunch with a dinner (linner, as one of my young patients calls it)—which is okay from time to time, as long as you're eating at regular intervals.

So, the time is late in the morning, just about lunchtime. This is an opportunity for you, the Weekend Warrior (next chapter, Chapter 6), to combine your two meals (saving some for your later-in-the-day half-meal). Can't you just visualize a lovely vegetable omelet stuffed with cheese and avocado and browned potatoes along with your fruit, and perhaps some skim milk in your coffee?

Personally, when I know I'm having a breakfast out in the later part of the morning, I eat a cup of yogurt topped with blueberries and a cup of decaf with almond milk at home as I'm preparing to go out. I don't go for long periods of time without refueling. So if I woke at six-fifteen a.m. and brunch isn't until twelve-twenty that's too long without fuel. Remember, you want to eat every four to five hours. Leaving room for hunger is dangerous because the *I don't care attitude* surfaces, and now your eating routine feels like a diet—which is what we're avoiding. Being too hungry leads to dangerous eating…

So get off the diet kick, and on to a simple formula that you can break down in any way that works for you, allowing you to travel or partake in any situation that presents itself. And now we're on to the Weekend Warrior mentality.

Personal Inventory Questions

1. It's summertime, or holiday time, and the diet mentality plus cheat day mentality is swirling something fierce. What to do? The temptations of dieting and bingeing are looming. Look back in time to your diet history. What was your first diet, and how did it impact you, and your relationship with food?
2. Magazines, perfectly displayed, are lined up to catch your eye, sporting the newest diet alongside a delectable dish loaded with a million calories. How does this affect you? Do you find yourself hopeful that maybe this one time a magazine article will do the trick?
3. Diet mentality is pervasive, chronic, and for some actually fatal. How does diet mentality affect you? Do you recognize it?
4. Do diets bring you happiness or cause you to feel slighted and cheated—that others can eat and you can't? And what about the new fads such as the keto diet or the weight loss surgeries that so many are tapping into, hoping *this time* something will work. Have you caught this diet train?
5. Lucas jumped on and off the diet bandwagon as far back as he can recall after his skiing accident on the slopes and

then student-abroad period. He searched high and low for the answer, missing the fact that he had a food addiction and needed to let go of certain foods before he could successfully release body weight. Do you have a similar story? Reflect on your earliest diets and how they've created a diet mentality in your life.

6. How about the idea of a formula to guide your eating? Do you think it's possible to plug in your food plan no matter where you go, or who you're with, or what's going on in your life? Do you have a formula?
7. Take the time to move those planned food groups around, creating lovely meals, rather than seeing the "formula" as a restriction. How does the idea of eating muffins or pancakes made from the five foods grouped in your morning meal sound to you? What mix of foods could you combine into a masterpiece?
8. Diets die, but creative food planning, with health-conscious, mindful eating in place, can free you from your diet mentality. What does this idea feel like to you? How about your creative juices coming up with a delectable breakfast at your favorite restaurant using the formula?
9. The idea of creating a formula is for you to organize your eating pattern in a health-conscious way that fits YOUR lifestyle. Eating a late breakfast can be a way to work in a brunch, combining a breakfast and lunch, as noted in the chapter. What are some ways you can design meals to fit your life conveniently, yet in a nutritious, healthful way?
10. When you visualize your plate of food, how can you combine foods in a way to make it most palatable for you? Food should be enjoyed, not just endured, but also meet your health needs.

Chapter 6

Weekend Warrior

We gain strength, and courage, and confidence by each experience in which we really stop to look fear in the face.
We must do that which we think we cannot.
~Eleanor Roosevelt

So you eat clean foods all week, feeling good about yourself, and then on the weekend all heck breaks loose. You say, *Oh but I've been good, it's my turn now. I want to enjoy the weekend and my friends are having a picnic*, or *it's my birthday*, or *my best friend is getting married*, or best yet, *You don't understand—I'm going on a long weekend getaway and I have to eat at Café Joe's because I always do and their cream blah blah blah is what I long for.*

Okay, I get it. Really I do. But this weekend warrior mindset is what gets you in trouble every single time. So, what's my version of the dangerous weekend warrior mindset? It's when you power through the weekend, starting on Friday and ending on Sunday, eating whatever you want because, well heck, it's the weekend. And *after* the weekend is over, a "come

Monday" kind of attitude resurfaces, telling you, *Okay, time to get serious.* You just had a cheat day on steroids leading to cheat daze.

A vicious cycle, don't you think? Is this a sequence you feel stuck in?

We gain strength, and courage, and confidence by each experience in which we really stop to look fear in the face. Do you want strength? Do you want courage? Do you want confidence? Then perhaps Eleanor Roosevelt's powerful words might be your go-to. *We must do that which we think we cannot!* Unless we eliminate worry and fear, or stare them down, implementing any strategy for success is very difficult.

You can go through a long weekend without diving into a vat of chocolate or whatever your food of weakness might be. *We gain strength, and courage, and confidence by each experience in which we really stop to look fear in the face.* You got this one. Abandon worry and fear, and you'll open a world of opportunity for both the inner and outer aspects of yourself—so that you *can* heal from the inside out.

Rocking to the Beat

Vivian hopped into her car, turned the ignition, and boom boom boom the radio blasted *"She loves you yeah, yeah, yeah. She loves you yeah, yeah, yeah"* from her Serius XM preprogramed Beatles Channel; as the convertible top slid into its slot, and she zoomed from first gear to sixth…*let the weekend begin.* Work had been intense, and now, brushing her hair out of her eyes as the breeze whipped into her face, she felt free. After all, work was grueling, and she deserved to let her hair down—so to speak.

Bobbing to the music— *"She says she loves you, And you know that can't be bad"*—as her car careened down the highway, Vivian felt free to enjoy four glorious days of nothingness. Singing and bopping, she felt as happy as could be, even though her innards twisted, and her head hurt from a stressed-out workweek. As if on autopilot, Vivian's car veered off to the nearest Publix grocery store so she could stock up for the weekend. *Ah the weekend!*

Up and down the aisles Vivian glided, filling her cart, grabbing steaks, chicken, vegetables, sweet potatoes…all the good foods…and then the golden bags of chips display nearly crashed into her cart. She stopped. Stared. And dreamt how good just one salty chip would taste—arguing in her head that she'd been so good all week, eating clean foods without messing up one inch.

Into the cart the chips went, and the doughnuts, and candy bars, and oh yes, what's a weekend without double-dip chocolate ice cream. Let the weekend warrior begin…

What happened! Where did Vivian go wrong? Her intentions had been good when she'd stopped at the store and began to fill her cart with all natural foods found in the earth, in the sea, off a tree. What went wrong?

First, she entered the store hungry since she hadn't eaten lunch because she'd had a late breakfast meeting and skipped eating, thinking that was a good thing.

Skipping meals is NEVER a good thing. When the tank drops low, we go into sloppy decision-making. Vivian walked into the store starving, tired, and really annoyed with her day, because a business deal had fallen flat at the last minute. She was ripe for the weekend-warrior I'm-going-into-eat-mode—which was the second part of her *going down*. The, it's-the-weekend mentality, meaning the *I deserve to eat bla bla bla* attitude, leads her down the rabbit hole every time.

Perhaps Vivian's story is your story, and you find yourself stuck weekend after weekend, messing up a beautiful clean week of eating. This is not uncommon. Heck the billboards and magazines, and the store itself, sends out signals, indicating this is the time for a food fest—a cheat day per se. The moment has come to eat, because it's the weekend, and parties, and family, and barbeques…and any excuse you can come up with.

Or, maybe you've been good all week with your food, but not your exercise, and you slip into another type of weekend warrior mindset that also leads you down the rabbit hole.

Exercise Warrior

Okay, so maybe you're not thinking of the weekend warrior time as an eating fest, but rather the weekend is your chance to exercise like crazy, to make up for the workweek when you didn't have the opportunity. You woke early and went to bed late, leaving no time to exercise. And your aim now is to work out. But then, after being pulled into the weekend eating frenzy, you have to dump the weekend warrior exercising plan with no time remaining to hit the stationary bicycle in the basement or the gym.

The goal of *Release Your Obsession with Cheat DAZE: Heal from the Inside Out* is for you to let go once and for all the long weekend excuse to eat what you want simply because it's the weekend, you deserve it, or that's just what you do—it's the weekend, *fa la la la.* Or it's the weekend, time for parties and friends, and FOOD AND DRINK. Instead, facing what you're up to as you read this book is about healing from the inside as you release your obsession with cheat foods because you honestly want to heal your lifestyle, body, misery, self-hate that arise when you eat without self-love.

But maybe you're the opposite. Maybe you're the weekend exercise warrior who can only exercise during the weekend, and you lay it on thick, thinking you can make up for the non-movement during the weekdays. This can turn into an exercise bulimia, something I'm all too familiar with.

Weekends, I'd ride my bike from my home to the Dania pier. Riding along the shoreline was lovely while smelling suntan lotion, hearing the laughter of walkers, and watching rolling waves crashing on the seashore. The outing was heaven—at first—but then it turned into three or four hours of weekend exercise, along with morning and evening exercise on the weekdays. My focus became a physical and mental excursion—a euphoric torture. But I *had* to, as I was making up for lost time—or so I thought.

But my weekend workout warrior mentality also linked itself to an eat-fest. I'd binge on whatever I wanted and then burn it off, too. I would power walk in the morning and bike ride with my husband at night. You might think exercising and moving my body to the point of exhaustion is not bad thing, but someone with exercise bulimia may find that they're sick more often than normal. Too much working out can weaken the immune system as well as make you prone to respiratory and other infections that a fatigued body may struggle to overcome.

People with exercise bulimia are obsessed with exercise and often binge. And rather than purging food on the spot, they instead exercise excessively as a way to lose the weight and relieve the guilt of bingeing. Cheat days led me to push my body, risking dangerous complications, including injury, depression, weak bones, and reproductive problems, and could have even lead to cardiac arrest. I was overusing my body—all to be thin—all to have my cheat days and be skinny at the risk of fatigue, pressure on my heart, increased miserable moods, muscle tears, etc.

Everything in moderation. Balance is the key to optimal health.

Batch Cooking…Line E'm Up

Maybe you batch cook for the week, utilizing the weekend to ready yourself for your workweek, but you also let yourself slip into being a passive eater during the weekend…because you've been so *good* all week. Batch cooking is an excellent measure to insure healthy meals throughout the week, but healthy eating is not an on and off option. It is rather a routine executed each weekday or weekend, holidays or vacation... You get the idea.

Eating healthy to bank for the unhealthy eating is not a helpful strategy.

This is the slippery slope we're trying to avoid at all costs. Every day should be business as usual when the question comes to your food and exercise. Yes, it's the weekend, and you deserve to have fun. But why do fun and food intertwine? When did you receive that message—and from where?

Wautoma Here We Come

Mom piled the six of us kids into her Chevrolet station wagon—ever so slick with the wood paneling on the side, and the power back window that opened so our feet could dangle out. My seat was all the way in the back…actually it wasn't even a seat, but a cozy place to set up the blankets and pillows for the long ride up to our cottage in Wautoma, Wisconsin.

Cuddles, our snow-white half-cocker, half-spitz, curled up next to me as the food fest began. Mom packed tuna sandwiches, chips, cookies, and soda pops for us to indulge in as we traveled the highway for four hours.

Debbie and I made sure to also have our stash of goodies that we'd bought from Penny's, the local candy store down the street. Our cherished brown paper bags were filled with red licorice for me and black for her, plus round, flat chocolates with white sprinkles, and saucers with candy dots inside (the texture always reminded me of communion on the tongue), and thick pretzel sticks covered in chunks of white salt. These goodies peeked out tantalizingly from the bag.

My idea of weekend, food, and fun was thus encrypted into my brain early in my life. Weekends meant food fest frenzy to me. I was a food fester—any festivity would do. Weekends meant family time, love, and freedom from school. Weekends imprinted in my mind that way as the happy time while weekdays were pure drudgery. Weekends equaled freedom—no pressure from the expectations placed on me.

What about you? What do weekends represent? The dictionary (dictionary.com) defines weekend as: "The period from Friday evening through Sunday evening, especially regarded as a time for leisure. It represents a time spent somewhere doing something—an expectation of fun, sun, and good times, all wrapped around food."

And the search begins, as we try to recapture a safe, fun moment in life that is murky at best. We confuse the emotion of feeling good with the food and the freedom of being out of school, or work, or perhaps both, and for me, headed to Wautoma, where the row boat awaits to capture any creepy-crawly, jumpy thing I could find in the water and bring home as my new pet, which was all the rage.

Tents were pitched on the beach, inviting late night swims, bonfires, and running barefoot—water skiing and horseback riding, all packed into a fun-filled weekend. The promise was set.

And the fun and love and freedom of no responsibility commingling with the warm and fuzzy sensation of eating sugary, carby foods became my craving. I learned early on that weekends were a time to eat, and a time to be free. I always felt trapped in school, as I watched the round, white-faced clock, with black wings pointing to the hour and the minutes, mounted on the wall, ticking away. I was mesmerized by the second hand twirling about, from 1 to 12; and then inching the long hand forward another minute.

I couldn't wait for three o'clock.

I stared out the window most of the school day, imagining and daydreaming of playing, running and jumping, and being free. Birds and white puffy clouds, with an occasional cat or dog meandering by, were my attention getters, as were the toddlers not yet imprisoned in school, laughing and playing and free. I so wanted to be free.

The Monday Through Friday Gig

Vivian also wanted to feel free. She felt trapped in her Monday through Friday job, glued to her desk, engrossed in the work task at hand, pausing from time to time, living for the weekend. The clock ticked ever so slowly before she'd be free to run, jump, and play. She too stared out the window, counting the minutes to freedom. She was not in a job she had a passion for, but loved the fact that she earned an amazing pile of money, week after week, and that she had an excellent pension plan of the type many longed for, as she was reminded of often.

Vivian was taught this was the way life was—that you worked and brought home money. Period. She never thought working a job with intention and filling your soul with a career of passion was possible, or even could be a reality.

Let's replay Vivian's scenario after a day of productive work. Though not all her deals went through, she did her best, and though this wasn't her dream job, she was respected and knew the ins and outs of her position.

Day after day she showed up at 8 o'clock sharp, often working as the sun set in an empty office, since co-workers left for home at the scheduled time. No, not Vivian. Though she was a clock-watcher, she also was an overachiever, buried in her job. Co-workers looked up to Vivian, who articulated and commanded attention when she spoke. Her words were calculated, and the results were amazing.

But solving and resolving consumer issues wasn't her life's calling. When she wasn't working, she read law cases, her true passion. Vivian was always told she didn't have the smarts for law, and that being an attorney was a man's work—and that she should be grateful for the job she had. So, she had settled for her current position.

Vivian lived for the weekends when she could be her true, authentic self, not boxed into a job she really did merely for the pay, not out of enthusiasm.

When she left work in the evening, Vivian was spent. Her frazzled self had a subconscious agenda of restoring her peace and tranquility that only a long weekend could bring. She indulged in weekends of booze and food, restaurants and bars, and hosting parties by her poolside with a bar completely stocked. But at the same time, she promised herself that the next weekend would be different. Nonetheless, week after week, come Sunday night, she'd know she'd overdone her "pleasures"—feeling bloated, lethargic, and most of all guilty.

Past Memories Morph into Present Memories

Vivian, the youngest of four children, had cherished weekends of family time, when Mom and Dad prepared lavish outdoor parties, with the Joneses and Smiths contributing side dishes. Kids ran free from house to house, jumping in and out of pools, the sun drying their little bodies while they drank from the water hose. And after all the scampering about, they were starving to eat all the delectables set forth on the patio and fill their hearts with the love and laughter all around them. Merriment and mirth rang out as the adults clinked glasses, swapping one story after the other. *And then it stopped.*

Vivian's dad took up with the secretary, Mom got a job, and the neighborhood gatherings ceased. Mom's job brought home a good income selling makeup, but sales wasn't her calling—just something she made money doing. Making money and keeping food on the table was the focus, and this mentality was passed along to Vivian. She took on the attitude that you can't count on a man to take care of you, that men leave you, that life is hard, and then you die.

And so Vivian's life became a quest to recreate childhood memories of merriment and mirth on the weekend and responsibility by weekday.

Heading to Publix, the wind blew Vivian's hair about as she belted out the latest Madonna song while making her mental list of what she was going to do over the weekend. She envisioned a lovely weekend of barbeques, walks on the beach, grilling seafood, and tossing fresh vegetables on the grill, all with the good intention of keeping up with her healthy eating she'd so precisely had in place all week.

Once in Publix, Vivian pulled out her list of foods she'd stored on her notepad in advance, knowing she was going to shop for the weekend. She knew from our work together that preparation was a key to beginning a long weekend without out-of-control eating. She'd agreed to choose wisely. Her list of *can eat* foods was far larger then the not-to-eat foods. She knew she had to stay away from sugar, flour, and wheat—that she must have nothing processed in order to be onto a perfect start of healthy eating, fun, and fabulous memories.

Vivian began with good goals, but she was hungry and frustrated, and longed for a weekend filled with the promise of joy. She unintentionally was trying to recreate her childhood memory of what a happy weekend presented, which was a family intact and friends filling the space with fun. Try as she might, that wasn't going to happen, because Vivian was single and didn't have friends to share the weekend with here as she'd just moved into a new neighborhood.

Self-love—Self-care

So, what's the answer? How do you move out of the weekend warrior mentality? Beginning with self-love and self-care by putting a plan in place gives you a good opening to dig in. You say, but Vivian *DID* have a plan—and yet her plan didn't work out. Well, yes she did have a plan, but what she had in mind wasn't set out with intention. Rather she was white-knuckling it with clenched teeth, with an *I'm gong to do this come hell or high water* attitude. That won't work.

Richard Carlson in his *Don't Worry, Make Money: Spiritual and Practical Ways to Create Abundance and More Fun in Your Life* suggests, "Being attached to an outcome, holding on, takes an enormous amount of energy, not only during an effort but often after an effort is complete, after you've failed, or been let down, or were dealt a bad hand." I began to read Carlson's book back in 1998, around the time I was standing in the kitchen with my mom chopping lettuce, and she blurted out, "Lisa, I think you have an eating disorder."

Back then when I was broke financially and healing from the inside out, and I was working on self-care and self-love, I recognized money and food often worked hand in hand. As I was becoming cleaner and clearer with my food and food addiction, I began to respect money along with my body, mind, and life.

I began to awaken, realizing if you hold on too tightly with food rituals (or money for that matter), you become too attached to the outcome. Simply let go of the outcome, as suggested by Carlson, and watch the change appear. The boomerang effect, he says, occurs when you abandon rigid rituals so that what you really are striving for pops up in doable, fun ways.

Trust the universe (or God, or whatever spiritual connection you might have)—and do your part—then let the idea go. When I was in Italy in 2016, I did just that. Though I had a formula, I couldn't always find the exact amount of food or in the order I preferred to eat—so I Let Go and Let God…only making sure whatever I did put in my mouth was real, unprocessed, and health promoting, and in as close to the right amounts as possible.

This approach worked!

I didn't walk around with inner diet chatter, cheat day mentality, shame, blame, or any self-judgment. I trusted my body and my food choices, bathed in my spiritual connection, and totally enjoyed the experience.

As Carlson says, nonattachment succeeds like magic. This way of living allows you to have fun in your efforts and to enjoy the process. In other words, letting go helps you succeed at whatever you're doing by giving you the confidence you need. Trusting life to bring you forward to the place you belong takes the pressure off. Vivian, on the other hand, went into the grocery hell-bent on stocking up on clean foods, only to cave at the first sighting of potato chips. All bets were off. She needed to get out of her own way. Instead of a tight grip, she needed to let go and trust that she could create a *healthy* weekend warrior mentality.

Create a Healthy Weekend Warrior Mentality

1. Stock and shop healthful foods on Sunday rather than Friday, when exhausted
2. Shop off your list only
3. Schedule weekend events that don't include food
4. Work in moderate exercise each day, not just on the weekends
5. Find quiet time to rest, read, meditate
6. Get a massage to release work-week stress
7. Plan social gatherings that don't revolve around food
8. Read a good book you can't put down
9. Write a book—share your story
10. Call a friend
11. Watch a movie sans the food
12. Find a place of worship if you practice a religion
13. Join an event and adventure group that doesn't revolve around food

14. Take a hot bath
15. Start a gratitude journal

A Weekend Escape

When writing this chapter, I was on a long weekend at my getaway place. My weekend consisted of walks along the beach, kayaking, and sitting in my swing overlooking the water. My meals started with my version of blueberry pancakes with a dollop of yogurt for breakfast; steak and roasted peppers for lunch; frozen peach yogurt for my half-meal; and then dinner—a succulent homemade coleslaw with chunks of chicken and peas rolled into a mayo/yogurt sauce.

Yes, oh yes I suffered on my weekend eating such delicious foods. No, eating healthy doesn't mean eating boring, but it also doesn't mean living to eat, but rather eating to live. And eating real foods that keep our bodies and minds, and our spiritual quests, intact. I am a weekend warrior, but in a health-conscious way.

My getaway once was a place where Mom and Dad gathered, clinking glasses and preparing luscious meals, but after Mom's massive stroke, and subsequent death, all gatherings stopped. For years, I tried to recreate *my* creation of those earlier family times by filling my belly with rich, processed foods, but as with Vivian, the results never came out quite as the picture I'd painted in my subconscious mind. In time, I learned to be present in the moment, rather than yearning for what once was.

Sure, the memory of those days is sacred, and I hold that time in my heart, but how things were was not quite the reality I sketched in my mind. My parents, for sure, were a misfit couple, though they loved each other in their own unique ways. My mom's last words to my sister were, "Tell Dad I love him." Though Dad worked and built a good life, in the end love is what's important in life, not the money, the achievements, the house, and the things. What's important is the love itself.

My father, to me, was bigger than life. He was famous in my mind. He could have been the accordion player for Lawrence Welk instead of Joe Feeny—the brother of Father Feeny, who I'll mention later on with an eerie connection, one to my father and one to my mother. Life does that somehow. But my father turned down playing with the Welk band as he didn't want to leave his family of origin—this was long before he ever met my mother.

My father also opened for Liberace—yes ***the*** Liberace—and can be seen in photos with President Nixon before Nixon's almost-impeachment. And Dad played for many important parties with influential stars and politicians. I recall one night he played to an audience including Leonard Nimoy—the *Star Trek* actor whose character had the pointy ears. I remember being wide-eyed, asking about those darn ears—only to learn they weren't real, though they sure were famous.

My mother, on the other hand, was a Katherine Hepburn sort to me. Not so much for her fierce independence and spirited personality, as exhibited by Miss Hepburn, but more in that she was a stunning beauty. My mom had good looks and a strong mind, and danced to her own beat, though she carried an enormous amount of weight in her adult years.

Mom loved horses, dogs, nature, and the outdoors. My father was the kind of guy who wore a bright-orange lifejacket when in a boat, and never walked in the sand nor ever held a tool or screwdriver of any sort. Yes, they were a mismatch—one a staunch Republican, while the other a Democrat—and I'm certain you can figure who was which. But they loved each other, in an odd sort of way—a Lucille Ball and Desi Arnaz kind of way. Dad, the musician dressed in a tux, attending gala events—polished and distinguished looking, and Mom gallivanting to her own shenanigans.

I took from each of my parents the good as well as the bad, but like Vivian, I eventually learned what I needed to do to make peace with my food and my food fest weekend warrior mentality. Vivian, to date, is living her best life, working at a law firm that fits her personality and needs. She attended night school and weekend programs at a law school near her job and began to build the life she wanted financially, emotionally, physically, and spiritually.

Vivian's weekend warrior is now no different than her weekday warrior, pursuing clean eating of three meals and one half meal, moderate daily exercise, drinking lots of water, and partaking in both rest and fun. She learned it's true that we gain strength, and courage, and confidence by each experience in which we really stop to look fear in the face. And, that we must do what we think we cannot, as Eleanor Roosevelt states.

Okay, so now that you have your weekend warrior mentality in check, let's take this mindset question a step further. What about *any* celebration excuse, as addressed in Chapter 7? Can you possibly enjoy the festivities without diving into an endless stream of food? Do you fear being caught up in the food fests frenzy so familiar during celebration time? Let's avoid the celebratory fog from cheat days as your jamboree begins.

Personal Inventory Questions

1. In what ways are your eating patterns similar to those shown in the chapter—that is, you start with good intentions, but find yourself bingeing? When did you first notice your weekends becoming a weekend warrior food fest?
2. What behaviors surface when you end your work on Friday night and begin your weekend? Do you see a pattern? Can

you identify the pattern and shift it to a healthy weekend warrior mentality?

3. What childhood memories surface as you think of your weekends when you were growing up? How do your childhood weekends impact you today?
4. I learned that we do, in truth, gain strength, and courage, and confidence from each experience, in which we really stop to look fear in the face. And, that we must do what we think we cannot, as Eleanor Roosevelt states. What are you doing that you thought you couldn't?
5. Vivian struggled during the weekends with food fest frenzy due to her childhood memories of what she thought fun and weekends meant. In time, she learned these images were merely illusions of what had been really taking place. Do you paint your childhood in a way that is more fabricated or embellished than your reality? How is that working for you?
6. What were your weekends like growing up? Are your memories of them fond or ones of loneliness? Did the weekends turn into a long food fest of uncontrollable eating?
7. What were your school years like for you? Did you live for the weekend or did you dread weekends? Why on either count?
8. Can you create a healthy weekend warrior list that will serve you during your weekends in a manner that makes the transition from weekdays to weekends blend together in a positive way?
9. What is your most cherished weekend memory, and what is your least favorite memory? Compare the two and see where one might blend into the other.
10. Every day should be business as usual in regard to your food and exercise. Yes, it's the weekend, and you deserve

to have fun. But why do fun and food intertwine. Where did you get that message?

Chapter 7

Any Celebration Excuse

You will find as you look back upon your life that the moments when you have truly lived are the moments when you have done things in the spirit of love.
~Henry Drummond

Dr. Wayne W. Dyer in a 2011 blog piece called Excuses Begone! said: *Learn how to change the self-defeating thinking patterns that have prevented you from living at the highest levels of success, happiness, and health by saying Begone—to all your excuses! You'll ultimately realize that there are no excuses worth defending, ever, even if they've always been a part of your life—and the joy of releasing them will permeate to your very core and you'll awaken to the life of your dreams.**

There are no excuses worth defending, yet for the food fester, any celebration excuse takes front and center. A food fester doesn't need a reason to eat, but put a celebration at the helm, and the eating frenzy takes hold. The celebration becomes the excuse to eat this or that, because, *heck, everyone else is, so why can't I, too?* This mentality says that these others, eating to their hearts' content, are having more fun and more joy, while you are harboring an attitude of deprivation.

But is defending the excuses worthwhile? Or would moving forward by releasing them be preferable so that you can reap the joy and awaken to the life of your dreams as Dr. Dyer suggests? Imagine the freedom to live your best life, not chained to the illusion: *This food will make me happy. If I eat this now, I won't do it again—I promise.* Or what about, *It's a holiday and not* ***realistic*** *to avoid eating those decadent desserts? What's a celebration without the good foods?*

If I could count how many times I've heard these excuses I'd be out of numbers. The most egregious defense? *It's not realistic.* This is the very one that will take you down that rabbit hole faster than you can say, "jackrabbit." Why? Because it leans toward "it's not fair," "it's not normal," "that's what everyone else is eating, so it must be the right thing for me."

Why is this line of thinking problematic? This excuse set is deeply flawed because the truth is that eating real foods ***is*** realistic. It ***is*** doable. And most important, these are foods from the earth that God presented for us to eat and sustain life. Release the wrongheaded excuses so you can reap your innate joy and awaken to the life of your dreams—the life of enjoying having a healthy body physically, emotionally, and spiritually.

Your Body Is a Miraculous Machine

Chalene Johnson, founder of the 131 Method, states, *Your body is a miraculous machine with self-healing mechanisms that in many cases you can activate simply through your nutrition.* Yes, that's what I've been saying to anyone who will listen. Our bodies are miraculously created, and we can each live life as healthy bodies, physically, emotionally, and yes, spiritually, healing from the inside out.

So how do celebration excuses work?

What is celebration? Is it the food? Is it the company? Is it the memory? And do you do these things in the spirit of love? Celebration is the action of taking one's pleasure at an important event or occasion by engaging in an enjoyable, typically social activity (Lexico.com). The key words in the definition are, "typically social activity" but for the eater, eating becomes the action to take one's pleasure, not the social event in and of itself. An eating frenzy is attached to the celebratory event.

Let's turn this around; eating doesn't have to take precedence. Let go of the eating focus, and concentrate on the event, the people connection, and gratitude, while placing food in the background rather than the foreground. Engage in the now, and stay present by listening and hearing what's going on around you, rather than becoming lost in the food that will soon take you into that numb abyss.

I'm certain that as you look back on your life, at the moments when you have truly lived, you don't recall the times you gorged on doughnuts, cookies, or rich foods in fat-laden sauces, but rather you think of the *moments when you had engaged in activities in the spirit of love.* Those are the times you truly lived. But somehow we forget that and look to a memory that's not quite real, turning it into our truth. Or worse, we don't remember at all because we were numbed out by the food taking over—or maybe even the drink.

I'm almost positive when you take your last breath before transitioning, you won't think or say, *Oh darn, I should have eaten the chocolate cake.* Perhaps you will embrace the loves of your life as you prepare to launch forward to greet your loved ones who have gone before you into the next step of existence. As I mentioned earlier, my mom's last words to my sister were, *"Tell your dad I love him."* And my mom was a food fester, of a different sort than I, but nonetheless a food fester. Why wait for your transition—or theirs—to connect and embrace?

If I Were Stranded on an Island…

I recall a talk I gave at a company known for producing luscious chocolates and savory cheeses, two foods that I'd consider my most favorites on the planet. In fact, as I began my presentation, I even became so bold as to say, *If I were stranded alone on an island and could only choose two items to tote with me, I would pick chocolate—dark and less than two grams of sugar—and cheese.* The group gasped—then roared with laughter.

They thought I was kidding—I wasn't. Those are two of my most favorite foods on the planet, chocolate and cheese, but I also know they aren't my *any excuse* to celebrate go-to foods. I remember what they tasted like, and in moderation, they're delightful, but they aren't my *everything,* nor are they my reason to be.

As I proceeded to discuss with the group my thought that if I'm stranded on an island, with nowhere to go—probably for the rest of my life—I might as well eat chocolate and cheese, until I transition to heaven. Excuse? Perhaps…but that's what we do. We make excuses for our eating behavior. Any excuse will do, even a justification as dire as being stranded on an island alone for the rest of one's life.

To think if such a tragedy happened that I'd want chocolate and cheese speaks volumes from a food addict in recovery.

At first, when I was summoned to give the talk at this lovely facility, I was asked to talk about diets, willpower, and commitment. As I thought about the topic, I considered that if I was to give an honest, authentic talk, then promoting diets would be moving away from what I teach.

I wouldn't be my authentic self, which I pride myself on being. My goal is to assist others on their journey to release their obsession with cheat DAZE—and to heal from the inside out, whether helping by way of this book, a blog piece, or in front of a group of people—so promoting a restrictive way of eating is moving further from the goal and surely to instill the obsession with celebratory eating.

Sometimes I'm misunderstood as being a diet doctor, especially since the name of my website is Weightcontroltherapy.com, not to mention the launch of my first two books: *Release Your Obsession with Food: Heal from the Inside Out* and *Release Your Obsession with Diet Chatter: Heal from the Inside out*—and now this third book in your hands. My offerings kind of look, on the surface, like those of a diet website or diet books—but I assure you they're anything but.

What are they?

I provide a website and two prior books (this is the third) on how to change your relationship with food. My approach begins with clean eating of real food. I ask readers to move away from garbage foods to glorious, natural foods, and heal—really heal— mentally, physically, and spiritually.

My goal has always been to present a rich and provocative understanding of chemical imbalance, psychology, and spirituality—a bio-psycho-spiritual point of view, as it relates to compulsive eating. And the bonus is weight loss. Hence the weight control therapy, and release your obsessions…all intertwining with the idea of creating a new relationship with food, so you can live your life like you've never lived your life—free and clear of food obsessions, regardless of the holiday, trip, long weekend, upcoming birthday, etc. These celebrations provide an opportunity to release excuses *so you can reap your innate joy and awaken to the life of your dreams.*

Therefore, I went back to the drawing board after a lengthy conversation with the human resources director who organized the event, and to my delight, a subtle switch was made in my talk topic to: ***Healthy Eating—Willpower—Staying True to Your Commitment!***

Ah…better, except the *willpower* part.

Willpower

What is willpower? It sounds like clenched jaws along with thinking: *I will not eat, I will not eat…I WILL NOT EAT!!!*

No, that won't do.

Willpower is right up there with diet…but let's see... How can I turn this around?

Let's start with healthy eating. What is that? Healthy eating is eating healthy. It seems simple, right? Nope. When I say eating healthy, visions of carrots, celery, and other types of "rabbit food" dance before everyone's eyes. Though those are delightful foods, the approach seems a bit diety. What about lovely homemade pumpkin muffins for breakfast with a dollop of vanilla yogurt, or coffee ice cream for a half-meal boost? Or how about chicken with French-fried sweet potatoes drizzled with coconut butter—air fried of course.

Okay, now were talking….

You see, we don't need any excuse to eat because eating is a natural and good thing and a necessity to sustain life. The *what* and *why* we eat are the topics that require closer examination. Healthy eating and nutrition become the focus, but understanding the what and why can get murky.

Why are you eating? Are you hungry, or are you emotionally craving to drown yourself in food? What are you hungry for? Do you want earth-grown foods with nutritional value or a high-calorie food with zero health benefits? Often, when someone is angry, crunchy foods are wanted; when the person is lonely, a creamy, sweet food is desired. All these desires are led by emotion. Yearning for a crisp salad with loads of colorful veggies, chunks of tuna topped with avocado oil and vinegar most likely is stemming from genuine, bodily hunger. So what you are eating can often lead to *why* you are eating—and such awareness is valuable in going forward.

Yes, healthy eating means eating nutritious foods—better yet, eating to sustain life—and a step beyond—what you eat determines how healthy your body is.

Today, the Standard American Diet consists of low fiber, high-fat processed foods. Not good. Nor is it healthy eating. Think of the acronym SAD. Yes, the Standard American Diet is sad—very sad, especially as it seems the norm.

Billboards, magazines, commercials, and internet pop-ups bombard us with gooey, chewy delights, letting us know that we NEED to eat these foods. And the advertisers often win. We make the excuse that we deserve that manufactured food, or staying away from those foods isn't realistic, or gosh everyone else is eating them, so why not me? Why do ***I*** have to eliminate these scrumptious foods while the happy, *thin* people are eating the foods in the advertisement? Look. They're smiling and swirling and having fun—*and they're thin.*

I want to have fun the way they are in the picture, you say to yourself. And, if I eat these foods, I will. SAD to think the standard American—me, and perhaps you—have been conditioned to believe these processed, non-nutritional foods are the acceptable ones. That the Standard American Diet consists of processed foods bought in fast food establishments—that cutting a fresh cucumber, tossed with spinach, kale, and tomatoes would be foreign to the standard diet of the American population.

Self-care is ignored, with people spending hundreds and thousands of dollars on foods that have almost zilch nutritional value. Think about what would happen if you bypassed the excuse to eat foods that don't promote optimal health and replaced them with store-bought produce and farmer's-market foods. You might be able to pocket the savings so that you could take that vacation, or enjoy a long weekend at a hotel near the beach, or city, or country, or wherever your fancy takes you.

Is the food really what we want—or what we feel the food represents? Our conditioning hypnotizes us to believe these foods will bring the party in the background of each advertisement into our lives. We don't consciously make this evaluation; we are lured into it through excellent marketing tactics. The job of the marketer is to convince the watcher, reader, listener, that this food will give us the happy satisfaction we are desperate to create in our own lives.

Excuses, excuses, excuses. The majority of people use the excuse they are too tired to make an elaborate meal, or that nutritious food may cost too much money. Hmmm, what does that sound like? Hmmm, is this an excuse, perhaps?

Healthy Eating

That healthy eating is costly, boring, or too difficult to put together is a myth. It's not. In fact, you can put a healthy meal together in less than thirty minutes. Sometimes waiting in line at the fast-food drive-thru can take thirty minutes from order time to pulling away from the window or the service counter. And for sure, making a home-cooked meal is much more cost effective than ordering takeout.

So what is healthy eating? Healthy eating is eating real foods that come from the ground, fly in the sky, swim in the sea, and come off a tree. Real foods are grown by nature—God's foods. They aren't in a box or a sealed bag or filled with preservatives. *Real foods will actually perish.*

Healthy eating consists of fruits, vegetables, starchy carbohydrates, dairy, fat, and—most important—protein. And if you visualize these natural foods combined, you can make homemade peach pancakes for breakfast or a raspberry coffee ice cream for a half-meal or stir-fried shrimp with colorful vegetables coated in garlic and olive oil for lunch. These meals become enticing, yet nutritious.

Combining the right ingredients takes a bit of creativity, and voila you are eating delectable foods that will contribute to your overall health AND give you the satisfaction you are yearning for.

Okay, I know you're stuck on the coffee ice cream, aren't you? What could this be? It's simple, and makes a perfect metabolic boost when you're ready for that in-between feeding after lunch and before dinner, or perhaps if dinner was served early, it makes for a perfect late-evening boost a few hours before bed.

Raspberry Coffee Ice Cream

One cup of plain, fat free Greek yogurt, one cup of raspberries mixed with one to two tablespoons (depending on strength preference) of decaffeinated instant coffee, a splash of real vanilla (sweetener optional) mix. Freeze until hard. And voila you have raspberry coffee ice cream.

Or, if you prefer, you could use unsweetened cocoa and pineapple instead of coffee and voila: chocolate-pineapple ice cream. Or, maybe you want a frozen-banana coffee ice cream. The exact ingredients are up to you. The choices are endless and satisfying, and most important, delicious *and* nutritious.

Healthy eating is eating foods that are palatable—delicious yet nutritious. That works.

What about that willpower thing again? Heck, who wants to be clenched-jawed, willing the self *not to eat*? Not me. Willpower is the control of one's impulses and actions: self-control. It manifests as a very strong determination to do nor not do something.

But as mentioned earlier, I often hear, *Oh no, I can't do that. It's not realistic.* What! Making a meal of real food isn't realistic? Why not? Our great, great grandparents and all the folks a few generations before us always ate real food. They didn't drive off to the nearest quick-fix joint to obtain their foods. No, they prepared it. And gave thanks.

But perhaps we're looking for an excuse for a cheat meal, food fest dinner. Eating out is an event. Eating fast food is an event. It's a party. It's easy. Yep, it's easy all right, until you find your clothes don't fit, you're short of breath, your joints hurt, and you really don't feel well. Ah, then the party you've been jonsing for—the celebration, comes to a screeching halt.

This isn't to say you can't eat out, because surely you can. And certainly you can choose foods that are packed with nutrients and even taste good. Stay away from the sauces and gravies and look for real foods that aren't processed, and you're good to go.

So, back to this willpower concept. Willing that you must do something isn't natural. Eating whole, real foods is. When we *will* something the action is not instinctive, it's almost like a stipulation, a rule. And human nature resists what we persist in doing—so rather than "willing" what we're going to do, how about accepting and embracing a new way of eating, so you can stay true to your commitment—the third part of my talk that day long ago.

How do you stay true to your commitment even if you're traveling, going on a long weekend, entertaining, or celebrating a holiday of some sort? You stay true when you accept and take ownership of your life.

Food Is Medicine

As I was preparing for my presentation, I stumbled upon an interesting article, by Dr. Sachin H. Jain entitled, "Sometimes Food Is the Best Medicine." Dr. Sachin admits he writes plenty of prescriptions for medicine to help his patients feel better but pondered over the thought of whether he could write a prescription for food. What a brilliant question. What if doctors prescribed *real food* as a medicine?

Real food—God's food—is often just the medicine we need. We look for a pill to make us feel this or feel that, when what we really need is food. Good food. Good old-fashioned grown in the ground, flying in the sky, swimming in the sea, hanging from the tree types of food. The kind of food, sans the chocolate and cheese, I might find on that island.

And if lucky, maybe a cow would be living there and a cocoa plant growing, and the island would be quite nice. No noise, but nature's natural sounds of birds tweeting, fish jumping, monkeys swinging from limb to limb. No internet, no television, no cell phone—just books, paper, and pencils. Sign me up!

Too often, we are unable to be true to our commitments because life stands in the way. Most of us are continuously plugged in. No escape. Our world, inner and outer, is noisy. Silence. Shhhh…listen to nothing. And then you'll begin to connect to the sounds of the earth. You'll be plugged into nature. For this very reason vacations are attractive to most of us. We are seeking to be unplugged—at least for a short time, before we start feeling as though we're missing out on something.

On one trip to Wautoma, my other paradise getaway, I was visiting with my sister Mickey. Wautoma, Wisconsin holds many dear memories together with some not-so-dear ones. Our vacation home is a place cherished by many generations back on my mother's side. Wautoma is a small town located in Waushara County with a population of around 1,500 people—a small place indeed. As children, we kids spent every summer there swimming, camping, skiing, horseback riding—as most of the tourists did during the nice weather season. After Labor Day, Wautoma becomes a quiet, quaint town without all the hustle and bustle.

Mickey and I still have delightful times together there as we both love our morning walks, eating breakfast out on the porch at the cabin in the middle of what feels like nowhere, enveloped by trees and near a small lake called Lake Mary (after my Aunt Mary of course!), and shopping for jewelry, in between going to Champion. Champion is the spot of a holy ground where apparitions of the Blessed Virgin Mary appeared on October 9, 1859 to Sister Adele Brise, who immigrated to the states from Dion-ke-Val, Belgium, and was instructed by the Virgin Mary to teach the children in the faith.

In the late afternoons we have our hot tea laced with almond milk and yogurt mixed with berries. Our time is sacred, but….

Are You Plugged In?

At some point, I feel the urge to plug in. Thinking back to one particular memory, I wasn't getting a signal out there in nowhere land, so I went by the trees, bending this way and that, trying to achieve a connection. Oh yes, I finally connected as I ventured deeper into the woods. I could hear my husband, Joe, saying, *"Hello, Lisa. Hello…are you there?"* Yes, I was connected to my husband, but if I took one step or swayed one inch, he disappeared. Looking down, I realized I was smack in the middle of a patch of poison ivy, and I heard the stirring of something BIG. I later learned bears now stroll through these parts. *Oh, but I was connected.*

We are so yearning to be plugged in. I just vaguely heard on the news about a woman who was trying to take a photo to post on social media, and she fell off a cliff to her death. And a man was walking and texting in a mall to the point at which he fell into a fountain. What we will do to log in online, yet we avoid the human connection at all cost. But that's another story for another book…

Unplugging, and eating healthy and nutritious foods, and having a glorious time on vacation is perfectly possible—and yes, you don't have to gain weight, or in some cases, depending where you are, lose weight. Let go of the excuses and tap into the reality of the now. *You'll ultimately realize that there are no excuses worth defending, ever, even if they've always been a part of your life—and the joy of releasing them will permeate to your very core and you'll awaken to the life of your dreams* (Dr. Dyer).

Traveling

When I travel, by car, plane, or train, I always bring my food, especially if I'm not certain if natural, untampered-with foods are available. I don't like to leave to chance that I *might* find healthy foods to feed my brain and body, especially when I'm headed to unfamiliar areas. Sometimes at amusement parks, libraries, airports prior to boarding the plane, or entering into other restricted facilities, I'm asked what's in the bag. Understandable, with all the shootings and horrific shenanigans, but after giving an explanation, I can usually pass through—except one time on an airline that restricted carrying more than a briefcase and a handbag.

I was stopped because I had my food bag as well. On that particular day, I stammered out my explanation of why I needed my food with me, and the attendant made me leave that bag behind. I became unwell on the plane. When the airlines learned why, they were aghast to think I was told I couldn't bring the food that I needed for my low blood sugar…hypoglycemic condition. Yes, you are might be thinking perhaps I needed a medical card, but actually you don't in most cases.

Now I know better. When asked what's in the extra bag I'm carrying, I say "my medicine." I have hypoglycemia and food is the remedy for preventing low blood sugar, which keeps me mindful of what I need to keep on hand at all times.

Food is medicine. In fact, Dr. Jain goes on to note a survey of doctors found that most wished they could write prescriptions for nutritious foods. This is very telling. The body operates at its optimal level when fed a wide variety of non-processed foods. We all probably have a touch of hypoglycemia if not refueling at regular intervals with natural mind/body food nourishment.

Access to nutritious foods is a game changer.

Real food heals the body of many ailments. Often my own patients come in with anxiety, depression, or some other combination of mood disorders, and on close look, the fact becomes apparent that they are eating processed foods with little to no nutritional value, leaving them agitated and unstable.

A Sugar Tantrum

I wrote an entire section in my book, *Release Your Obsession with Diet Chatter: Heal from the Inside Out* about Baby Jessica, a toddler sucking on a gooey frosty drink grasped with chunky fingers, weighing as much as if she were five years old. She pulled a complete temper tantrum in my office to the shame and embarrassment of her mother, who actually had come to see me due to weight gain shortly after her weight-loss surgery.

Mom's old habits began to resurface because she felt she was *missing out* on her food fest frenzy and she had returned to her old pattern of eating. On this particular day she had to bring Baby Jessica because the babysitter bailed due to Jessica's usual temper tantrums.

I love children, and make it known, even on this particular day. How bad could Baby Jessica possibly be? Sticky-fingered, wide-eyed Baby Jessica began pulling, climbing, and grabbing anything and everything within her reach as her cherry slurpy spilled every which way. When she attempted to climb up on the window frame wooden slats, they came crashing down, and shortly after, she plunged her fingers into the fountain neatly tucked in the corner of my room—once she'd poked her fingers into the oil lamp near my chair.

Mom scolded red-faced Baby Jessica, who fell to the floor, kicking and screaming as loud as her little lungs could take her until she fell fast asleep, at which time Mom and I had a serious discussion about food and mood. Mom's excuse was she didn't have time to cook real food and that her children deserved to food fest like the rest of the planet. But after a while, we made great strides in our discussion until the little one stirred awake, frantically looking for her red slurpy, and the saga started all over again.

I'm pleased to say Jessica, now in middle school, weighs a healthy number, and is composed and well adjusted. Mom and family made a complete turnaround in their moods after releasing their obsession with the food fest frenzy mentality, and their food consumption is no longer upside down—after a complete shakeup.

Out with the junk food, and in with the nutritious, delicious real foods.

Jessica's husband no longer needed anger management classes, and her son was able to let go of his Adderall for attention deficit disorder. Baby Jessica turned into a lovely, poised, delightful girl. And the mom, she lost excess weight—as did the entire family, and all is well, which brings me back to the third point of my talk which is ***staying true to your commitment***.

Stay True to Your Commitment

Staying true to your commitment means omitting diet mentality, junk food, and excuses to celebrate with food, and turning instead to daily lifestyle overhaul—eating real foods with nutritious value.

Food is medicine.

Every food eaten should serve a purpose such as feeding your cells, brain, and all other essential organs, not to mention creating clean blood.

A successful change of eating habits revolves around healthy eating, and instead of willpower, we switch to willingness for change and most importantly, staying true to our commitment. When what we eat is NOT a diet, but a change in lifestyle, that allows our commitment to last a lifetime.

Lifestyle change means exercise, healthy foods, sleep, water, relationships, and a playtime work-time…balance.

So, do diets really work, or are they a never-ending promise to deliver an option that doesn't really exist? The answer is easy, diets die; they are temporary rather than lifelong.

So, off I went to speak to an impressive company that makes chocolate and cheese—my two most favorite foods on the entire planet and delved into excuses followed by solutions.

Excuses take hold in all forms—even with the loss of a loved one. Excuses can blend into grieving and loss as an attempt to fill the emptiness. Part II, Realignment, directs us to Chapter 8, where we'll explore the loss of a loved one, which is inescapable and inevitable in all of our lives.

Personal Inventory Questions

1. Is it possible *you'll ultimately realize that there are no excuses worth defending, ever, even if they've always been a part of your life—and the joy of releasing them will permeate to your very core and you'll awaken to the life of your dreams?* Do you make excuses for why you need to eat this or that? As you read Dr. Dyers quote on excuses, what came to mind?
2. It's not uncommon for me to receive requests to speak about diets. As noted, when diets were *almost* a part of one particular presentation of mine. What are your thoughts about using "diets" to motivate you to lose weight?
3. What is celebration? Is it the food? Is it the company? Is it the memory? And do you embrace these elements in the

spirit of love? Celebration is the action of taking one's pleasure at an important event or occasion by engaging in enjoyable, typically social activity (Lexico.com). What comes to mind when you hear the word "celebration"?

4. I'm certain that as you look back on your life that the moments when you have truly lived you weren't eating doughnuts, cookies, or rich foods in fat-laden sauces but rather the *moments when you had undertaken activities in the spirit of love*. What have you done in the spirit of love?
5. When I was presented as a guest speaker recently, I became bold enough to say if I were stranded alone on an island and could only choose two items to tote with me they would be chocolate—dark and less than two grams of sugar—and cheese. What two items would you choose to bring with you?
6. At first, when I was summoned to give the talk at this lovely facility, I was asked to speak about diets, willpower, and commitment. Which of these three resonate with you and why? Delve deep, pulling from your personal experiences to learn the whats and whys of your excuses.
7. What is your definition of healthy eating? Do you eat healthfully, or does it leave you with a bad taste (no pun intended). Do you employ willpower in your healthy eating plan? Do you find willpower is needed to shape your thinking?
8. What family genetic played into your relationship with food? Did your mom freely give you junk foods at an early age like Baby Jessica?
9. Is it possible food can work better in some cases than prescribed or over-the-counter medicines? What are your thoughts about doctors prescribing food in addition and/or instead of medicine?
10. Sometimes, amusement parks, libraries, or airports prior to my boarding the plane, will ask what's in my bag. Do you

refrain from bringing your foods with you for fear of getting into trouble? How do you work around that?

* Dr. Dyer was also the author of the 2009 book *Excuses Begone!: How to Change Lifelong, Self-Defeating Thinking Habits.*

Part II

Realignment

Chapter 8

Loss of Loved Ones

What matters in life
is not what you're busy doing or having,
But what you're busy BEING.
Whatever you ARE
is what you will experience in your life.
Your 'beingness' equals your life experience.
~Soren Lauritzen, the Personal Development Guy

People come and people go—an inescapable rhythm of life. Though death is inevitable, the potential or real loss of loved ones is often concealed far back in the recesses of our minds, perhaps too painful for some to look at head on.

An Internship Gone Right

Earning my Master's degree in social work with an emphasis on mental health came with the responsibility of seeking two internships. After a long search, I settled on two completely different experiences. The first was at Sylvester Cancer Center, working with patients in the terminal cancer ward, and the second was at Jackson Memorial Hospital's psychiatric ward.

Sylvester Cancer Center taught me more about dying—and living—than any course or event in my entire life.

At Sylvester, death was imminent. Every person there was in the process of transitioning. Inside nearly every door I passed through, I was greeted by a baldheaded patient stripped down to their bare self—their authentic self.

To be honest, I was *not* looking forward to this internship; it came out of nowhere. I was leading a Weight Watchers class at Jackson Memorial Hospital in Miami when a participant, Judy, heard I was in school and that soon I needed to secure an intern position.

At the time, they had no interns on this particular ward, but Judy insisted she could open the position, and supervise me. I wasn't at all interested. I wasn't a fan of death and dying, hospitals, wounds, or anything of the kind. In fact, in high school I nearly passed out at the hospital during our health and CPR training class, due to my aversion to tubes, blood, and whatever else.

I took the assignment.

I learned more in that internship than I ever imagined, and the dreaded experience turned into a blessing that has guided me through all of my days to this very moment. My takeaway was: People who live their best lives doing the work they love; living with people they love; balancing fun, play, family, and work; and who have a connection to a higher source—whatever that might mean to each individual—seemed more at peace while dying. I found patients who had lived—really lived—moved through the dying process with the most grace and dignity.

Not one person was about food or eating for entertainment. True, appetite changes at the end-stage of life, but *nobody* made food their focus, which at the time was foreign to me as I was knee deep in my cheat days and over-exercising drama.

Annie Embraces End of Life

I recall a lovely eating-disordered patient, Annie, I worked with many years ago, years after my Sylvester internship, who called me from the clinic where she'd had a routine exam. I was her second call. *"I've got the Big C."* My heart sank. I continued to listen with the phone pressed tightly against my ear as she was speaking almost in a whisper. She embraced her news with strength and dignity. Although certainly not everyone diagnosed with cancer dies within a short period of time, due to the particulars of her situation, I well understood the course she was on.

Annie marched forward with great courage, ready to transition from this world to wherever the next stop would be. The only fear I ever knew Annie to have was fear of being overweight. She had been haunted with extra pounds most of her life, but now, for the first time ever, she could eat whatever she wanted—*and yet she had no interest in food.* The irony, was all the foods she *thought* would make her happy never did. The events in her life were what made her life.

The last time I saw Annie was at the home of her daughter, Macy. Annie insisted Macy pull out a pint of chocolate monkey something. We giggled at the name and at the glint in her eyes, and her mischievous grin, as she dove in to eat for the first time without guilt. The sad part was she couldn't really eat this formerly forbidden food. Two bites, and she was set. Annie passed shortly after. From her diagnosis to her passing took six weeks.

My heart hurt when I learned of Annie's passing. She was a delight to work with, always kind and gentle, and with a ready smile.

When we lose a loved one, the pain is undeniably deep. Those who lived full lives of *being*, though, are sent off without a heavy heart. Knowing someone lived each moment to the fullest is the ultimate. Annie chased the *thin* dream all of her life, and only began to experience thin a few months before her diagnosis—not realizing she was already quite sick. I recall her swirling around in my office, pulling on the waistband of her pants, saying, "Look I'm getting so skinny" with a big smile spread across her face. This was before she learned of her cancer.

Annie was accepting and open to her diagnosis, as well as the thought of transcending to the other side. Her funeral was a celebration of her life with all her beloved foods and pastries spread out for a banquet.

But no doubt that pain of a death cuts like a knife for those who remain—they feel an emptiness. Emptiness, often filled with something, whether booze to numb, or food to fill the hole, or drugs to escape the reality.

And Then Delanie

Delanie, the first girl born after seven brothers, the apple of her father's eye—a mini version of her mom, grew up in a warm, loving Catholic family. Being the only girl, and the last child at that, she was put on a pedestal. Life was laughter and joy, and fighting too. You see Dad often came home from a long day's work, staggering his way up the steps, muttering nonsense as he found his way to the couch. And the brothers, not too far removed from Dad's imbibing, began dabbling in this drug or that early on in life.

Mom (Patricia) found her way to the chocolate doughnuts and fried goodies to fill her heart from the not-so-fun times in their home. When life was good, it was very good, but when it was bad, it was awful. But, as our tendencies go, the good often is glorified, and the bad gets tucked away as the family secret, not to be told.

One stormy night, as Hurricane Andrew, a category 5, struck the Bahamas, Florida, then Louisiana, in mid-to-late August of 1992, all braced for what was yet to come. The sun was out that morning, not a cloud in the sky, as the father, Sean, and his buddies sat in the local Irish pub sipping on cold draft beer, watching as The Weather Channel blasted the latest tracking information for the storm pummeling through the Bahamas on that balmy August 23rd, soon to make its way to South Florida.

When the wind began to stir, Patricia, Delanie's mom, directed each family member to begin the process of boarding up the home while she and Delanie bought food supplies, and what is known as "hurricane food," as everything began to still, and the sun disappeared, replaced by large, thick, black clouds. Birds fluttered this way and that, and the Atlantic began churning, tossing boats to the side like toys. One by one, the teen boys returned home to organize and prepare.

Dad made his way home while the wind picked up, and drops of rain began to fall. The guys began slowly and methodically to put up perfectly measured sheets of wood, covering one window at a time. Delaney and Mom filled the bathtub with water, along with empty jugs and ice cube trays, knowing soon the power would cut off, and they'd be in the dark.

In the wee hours of the morning, hunkered down, waiting for the storm, the guys drank, and Mom and Delanie delved into the "comfort" food supply. Huddled with the battery-operated radio, they listened to the now-famed voice of weatherman Bryan Norcross, who became known as a steady and reassuring, calming voice when the winds howled, and sounds of debris tossed about could be heard.

The family pulled together the way they always did in times of need, doing what they had to in order to protect each other. Sean, concerned after a loud crash, wanted to see what had happened, in spite of his wife's plea to stay in until it was over—as instructed by the weatherman—the only voice they'd clung to throughout the night. But in his typical stubborn fashion, Sean went out with Keith, the oldest son: neither ever to return.

Silence replaced the laughter once heard in the Riley home, each turning to a substance of choice to cover the pain…but no food, liquor, or drug could fill the stillness—the broken hearts. In time, of course, the family went on. Life goes on, broken or healed, from tragic events. This family turned a corner, healing and mending, pushing forward.

Death, illnesses, and divorce all can lead to out-of-control eating, drinking, drugging, shopping, but the pain only intensifies with the numbing. The Rileys began to embrace and cherish life, leaning on their Catholic faith and family unity. Rather than remaining broken, they mended and celebrated Keith and Sean's lives, never forgetting, but instead, going on to live, believing their loved ones were close by watching over them, and that one day, they too, would join them in the beyond.

The Wind Whirls and Hurls…

That same night Hurricane Andrew touched many other lives, including my own, though not as tragically as those of the Rileys. I was huddled with my then-inebriated husband, my toddler, and others who I can't recall. My sister-in-law, someone I adored, was forced to go to the hospital as she was a high-risk pregnancy patient in her late term, leaving me alone with the intoxicated men.

I, too, clutched the radio, listening to the wind whirling and slamming whatever stood in its way, while the calming voice of Bryan Norcross comforted me in the dark as I held onto my baby.

I was terrified.

We, too, had bought supplies—and yes "hurricane foods," which consisted of fried chicken, chips, doughnuts, candies, water, and more water...jugs and jugs of water. And don't forget the soda pops, beer for the guys, and bread with different sliced meats. We had ingrained in us the idea of making sure to have nonperishable foods, so cans and cans of foods also lined the pantry shelves.

Many throughout the area, and still to this day, conduct hurricane parties. It's an event! The grocery stores and hardware stores become overcrowded with shoppers and shelf after shelf in the groceries is stripped of every nonperishable food. Tempers flare as lines form in the stores, not to mention lines around the blocks and horns blowing as people impatiently wait for gas.

The night of Andrew was a long, long night.

Though my home didn't suffer the devastation of collapsing like a house of cards as did residences further south in Homestead, trees and debris fell on our house, cutting the power for three weeks. Though I was in denial, my marriage was unraveling at the seams while my husband's alcoholism and my food addiction were in full rage. I was in the process of grieving my own losses: the loss of family and the dream of a solid marriage and the hope of growing old together. I was in sorrow over what was not going to be—a mother, father, and children, whole and intact.

Many lives were lost that night, and homes demolished by high winds, rain, and tornadoes that were soon to follow. Exiting our dark space after calm resumed was like coming out of a cave and entering a battle zone after hours upon hours of being shut in with windows blocked so that no light of day could be seen.

Lives change as losses mount. But we can embrace and move forward, or we can let the grief take us down.

Death and Dying

Early in my undergraduate years, I learned about Elizabeth Kubler-Ross, a Swiss-American psychiatrist, who in her 1969 book entitled, *Death and Dying: What the Dying Have to Teach Doctors, Nurses, Clergy, and Their Own Families,* taught about the five stages of grief, also known as the Kubler-Ross model. Though originally this model was patterned for grief stages of the dying, it morphed into a representation that is plugged into many scenarios of grief and loss. The five stages chronologically are: denial, anger, bargaining, depression, and acceptance.

The Rileys were in total shock when Sean and Keith never returned that stormy night, at first believing and yearning that they would. Believing someday the two would come home, returning to the laughter and loud fights, to which they all were so accustomed.

Patricia was angry to lose her husband and son—angry with God for such cruelty. She begged God to make this be not so, that she'd be a better wife, a better mother, but days of silence ensued. The once-lively home was no more. Patricia drifted into a deep depression, back and forth between the different stages, until she made her peace with what had occurred and accepted life's twists and turns.

In many cultures, death is celebrated, with the mourners knowing that the person returned to God. Rather than having a funeral, they hold a celebration of life. That event is one of celebration of *being* and a celebration of loved ones moving on to a better place with the angels and connecting to those close ones who had passed before.

Foods of all sorts are prepared and served. A last sacred meal is shared among friends and family swapping memories.

Food fest frenzy with high sugared, high-fat foods doesn't have to adorn the tables to recreate stories of a life well lived. A spread of fruits, fish, chicken, meats of sorts with an arrangement of colorful vegetables to start can create a healthy, spiritual event, with natural foods of the earth prepared in an unprocessed way.

My parents both passed on Thursdays—and each time I didn't make it to be with them for their final breaths, but I recall experiencing the pain of loss, rather than dodging and numbing with food or substances as I once might have done.

On a Thursday evening, only hours after my mom's transition, arriving from Florida, I stayed at her home that Dad had purchased and cleared, making it into a space where we could care for her during her last four years of life, paralyzed after a stroke. It was a makeshift hospital, but with the kitchen nearby she could observe and direct any cooking. A fireplace kept her warm, and she enjoyed a lovely view out the window of birds feeding off the feeder my brother Danny set for her to see.

That first evening, I slept in my dad's bed, as he never returned to that home again. Preparing to lie down, doing my nightly grooming, I opened a drawer in the bathroom, and to my surprise, I found the last bottle of mom's Valium. I held the bottle, staring at the label for what seemed like hours, debating whether I should take one of the remaining pills. I didn't. While I didn't want to accept that her life was over, and I didn't want to believe she was gone never to return, I nonetheless slowly, in a trance-like state, placed the bottle back where I found it. I returned to bed, allowing myself to feel rather than numb myself out.

Letting go of loved ones is never easy, especially if feeling your feelings is challenging to begin with. I'm grateful for the four years with my mom before she passed away, as we shared many laughs—and frustrations too. Kubler-Ross's five stages of grief applied to me, the living, as much as they do to a person diagnosed with a terminal illness, someone who has an accident leaving them disfigured, a person whose marriage ends abruptly like mine or like Patricia's, or one suffering the loss of a loved one after years of care for an illness. Each person may well go through denial, anger, bargaining, depression, and finally acceptance.

After her stroke, my mom became more demanding and difficult than she had been, and she lost her ability to feel any emotion due to her right hemisphere injury, which impacted her left side leaving her paralyzed with impulsive behavior and mood changes. She had trouble paying attention or resolving basic situations. Mom also had a fear of falling, though she was unable to move or to roll.

Her passing after a long and debilitating convalescence should have been a relief to the family, but I was angry. I was angry because my mom died in her sixties and had so much more life she should have lived—and grandchildren to watch grow and marry, and even have children of their own.

I was depressed because I was gypped of time with my mother and had bargained that if she could just get better…denying this was the way it was going to be. That she wasn't going to walk ever again, or drive, or show her well-known German shepherds, winning champions sought throughout the country.

But in time, after years of swaying from one stage to another, I began to experience what Ms. Ross describes in her book, that rather than our shying away from the "hopelessly" sick, getting closer to them can help them during their final hours. The few able to do this will also discover that the experience can be mutually gratifying; they will learn much about the functioning of the human mind and the unique human aspects of or existence, and will emerge from the relationship enriched and perhaps with fewer anxieties about their own finality.

And I think time spent with my mother during her last four years did just that for me. I already had begun to understand life and death tied to spiritual awareness and acceptance of transitioning from my time at Sylvester Cancer Center. I learned from each patient facing their life coming to an end—that death is inevitable.

I learned what living a full life meant. I learned to accept death with an open heart. I learned that sitting and listening to another with love and an open heart is the greatest gift we can give one who is preparing to transition.

And their stories helped me to reckon with my own ageing process and ultimate, impending death. To live life to the fullest NOW is the quest of many who have been blessed to make peace with death and dying.

Events, whether a death, divorce, break-up, a difficult move and so on, don't have to revolve around food to fill the pain, but rather require foods to feed the brain, emotions, and every part of our being. No need to numb ourselves with sugar-laden foods, or any substance, as this won't take away the pain. The real resolution of the pain comes from moving through the pain, rather than burying it. We will be blessed when we face the reality head on. And celebrating the life of a loved one—sharing precious memories—is the greatest sendoff you can give another.

Turning from endings to living, and accepting life, and how we might face what's eating us, rather than what we're eating is up next, in Chapter 9.

Personal Inventory Questions

1. What matters in life is not what you're busy doing or having, but what you're busy BEING. Whatever you ARE is what you will experience in your life. Your 'beingness'

equals your life experience (Soren Lauritzen). So looking past what you're doing, ask yourself: What is your 'beingness' and how does it factor into living your best life?

2. Sometimes in life we are thrown into a situation we didn't plan or expect—and we have to face our fears. I wasn't looking forward to my internship at Sylvester Cancer Center. Were you handed an experience that pushed you to do something you really didn't want to, but in hindsight realized the blessings it brought into your life?
3. Annie fearlessly received her news that she had cancer and greeted her death with total acceptance, moving through each step as if it were a normal path of life—and it is. Do you know of someone like Annie, and if so, how did that person's situation impact you and your relationship with death and dying?
4. Unfortunately, natural disasters such as Hurricane Andrew are unavoidable, and can do harm, and even take lives. Delanie lost her dad, and brother as the storm went through. Rather than giving up on life, the family, after their natural grieving process, began to thrive, making life count. Perhaps you've undergone something heartbreaking such as this family, or you know of someone who did. What was the takeaway for you?
5. In many places prone to hurricanes, the oncoming disaster often morphs into "hurricane parties," with junk foods of all sorts. This comes from a *what the heck* or end-of-the world attitude: It's going to storm and harm could come our way so we might as well eat. What do you think about that? How will eating the foods impact the consequences of the storm?
6. Storms, tornados, widespread fires and such can change the course of a population's life with losses or devastations of entire areas. Coping can be challenging, or it can open new opportunities. What has been your experience, and

how have your grown or lost personal headway from it? What would you do differently if anything, if you had to face the same situation again?

7. Elizabeth Kubler-Ross, a Swiss-American psychiatrist, in her 1969 book entitled, *Death and Dying: What the Dying Have to Teach Doctors, Nurses, Clergy, and Their Own Families* defines the five stages of grief, also known as the Kubler-Ross model. The five stages chronologically are: denial, anger, bargaining, depression, and acceptance. Can you identify with these stages?
8. Sometimes in life we lose family members early, leaving an emptiness marked so many times by events such as weddings, graduations, birthdays, and such. If this is your case, how have you moved through these occasions without making them a food festivity to cover the pain of the loss? Do you think you could avoid eating out of control in such an instance?
9. How does your family culture view death and funerals? Do you engage in a celebration of life or do you move through the funeral process in a more solemn manner?
10. How do you view death and dying? Do you spend time thinking about it or brush the thought away? And in either case, how is that impacting your life?

Chapter 9

What's Eating You?

The truth is that
there is no actual stress or anxiety in the world.
It's your thoughts that create these false beliefs.
You can't package stress, touch it, or see it.
There are only people engaged in stressful thinking.
~Dr. Wayne Dyer

Okay, let's think about all the focus on ***this*** diet and ***that*** diet—to eat ***this*** and not to eat ***that***. But what if the real concern needs to be not about what you eat, but rather what's eating you? Could something be going on within that has nothing to do with food?

What about stress? Dr. Dyer says the truth is that we have no actual stress or anxiety in the world—that we can't package, touch, or see it. He's suggesting stress is something we're creating in our mind.

I speak about the mind and its stories at great length in my second book: *Release Your Obsession with Diet Chatter: Heal from the Inside Out.* And with *this* book, I'm looking at the thing we do when we go into "vacation mode" and turn to food for fun, happiness, freedom, and whatever else we imagine this food fest frenzy will bring to us. Sadly, though, our vacation mode scramble for food as the event is a cover-up for what's really going on. Often this type of "vacation" thinking meanders to the cheat day mentality—just because.

A Man and His Best Friend

As I prepared to write this piece, I received an unexpected email from a patient we'll call Nikko, who I see once a year around Christmastime, just for a check-in. Nikko has blossomed into a lovely thirty-something young man, growing out of the insecure, lanky teenager who felt disconnected from the world.

I was surprised to hear from Nikko, as the month was barely June, a long time off from Christmas. These days Nikko is a travel writer who makes his way around the world writing about this adventure and that adventure. He always was a free spirit, even as a young teen when we worked together revealing his true, authentic self.

Nikko dreamed of traveling and writing, and having a dog companion by his side everywhere he went.

And he did just that.

Nikko traveled with Bruno, a crazy, loveable, chocolate Labrador who melted every heart he slobbered wet kisses on.

This particular June day when Nikko came into my office, he sported dark circles under his eyes, his frail body hunched over, walking as if he were elderly. This was not the Nikko I knew. Nikko had been through many bouts of different cancers in his young life, weathering and powering through each one like a trooper, always upbeat, and living in the moment. But today he was off. I feared the cancer was back, and maybe he wasn't going to beat it this time.

But Nikko's story that day turned out to be about Bruno. His best buddy who had always been by his side—*and I mean always*—was gone. At first, I didn't know what to say, and I'm not one to stammer and be at a loss for words—or emotions for that matter—but when the topic comes to animals, my heart goes to mush.

In one of those unexplainable incidents, Bruno, out of nowhere, had respiratory problems and couldn't breathe, to the point where Nikko had to perform mouth-to-mouth resuscitation. But to no avail, as the dog died in his arms.

Yet Dr. Dyer says the truth is that we have no actual stress or anxiety in the world—that we can't package, touch, or see it. He's suggesting the emotion is something we're creating in our minds.

Did Nikko create in his mind that Bruno died unexpectedly in his arms? No, of course not. Nikko, for sure, was not simply creating anxiety and stress in his mind. What he was experiencing was real. He was working the process of letting go of his best friend, and the hole in his heart was painful—and it ***was*** real.

Nikko was grieving. The loss of Bruno was the unexplainable, and outside of him and his control. He knew what was eating away at him. His suffering wasn't about food, or weight, or girls, or travel, but about loss—a vacant space in his life. A best buddy, who loved unconditionally—no matter what—was gone.

We have to deal with such life blows before we can eventually find our way to acceptance and a release of stress. Only then we can understand Dr. Dyer's point of view that stress and anxiety aren't inherently part of the world.

I understood Nikko's loss all too well, as but three years before, I'd lost my precious Sage, a white Swiss shepherd we had rescued. She was always near at hand, resting her chin on my foot as I wrote my first book (*Release Your Obsession with Food: Heal from the Inside Out*)—with me every step of the way.

Sage was there when my mom died, our son left for college, and I was awarded my Master's then my doctorate. She was my best friend. And when she was struck with degenerative myelopathy (DM, a spontaneously occurring, adult-onset spinal cord disorder that affects dogs—and is similar to amyotrophic lateral sclerosis, ALS or Lou Gehrig's disease in humans). With DM, the dog suffers a degeneration of the "white matter" of the spinal cord and the peripheral nerves.

Very gradually, Sage became paralyzed. At first she'd fall down for no apparent reason…and at the end, she couldn't stand at all. We clung on to her longer than we should have and then called the vet to come to our home and help with her transition the day after Christmas. The night before, our older boy carried her outside onto the patio and washed her, sobbing. Just thinking of it still brings tears to my eyes.

So yes, I felt Nikko's pain deeply—and his pain wasn't about what he was eating but it *was* about what was eating at him, to the very core of his being.

So, what's eating *you*? Is the food your real problem, or is something deeper digging into you? Are you missing your passion? Or is your sorrow about not having a direction to your life and that your current path has lost its luster?

Is Stress Lurking or Is Fear Knocking?

Maybe your issue isn't what you're eating at all, and it is about what's eating you. Could your difficulty be stress, or possibly fear, or how about maybe missing your true passion in life? I hear all too often from patients that they don't know what they're meant to do—that they don't have a real passion to pursue. They've become paralyzed with fear of not knowing why they're here on this earth, questioning their *calling*.

Fear is a motivator to focus on something other than what's really bugging you. Not uncommonly, those in my field, working with eating-disordered patients, learn these individuals have a fear of growing up; so to distract from this worry, they put their focus on the food, or the exercise, or some type of purging behavior.

I recall one patient, Ally, who stopped eating so she could have a boyish body with no curves, thinking this would keep her a child. Yes, she looked fifteen years old when in fact she was closer to thirty. But her strategy wasn't working for her, since she was, in actuality, an adult with all its attendant trials and accountabilities. Ally became depressed to the point of not wanting to live.

Together, she and I looked her fear smack in the face. Ally, relying on therapy and self-analysis, came to terms with what was happening with her both internally and externally. She learned, as adults, we can't defy ageing, growing, accepting responsibility, and living an adult life, if we are to truly live.

I've also seen a host of other patients harbor intense fear of success—or worse, what about the fear of no clue what to do with an entire life—which is a mighty long time. Often I hear patients say, *"I should know what I'm doing because so-and-so knew when he was a little kid."*

I Want to Be a Monkey When I Grow Up

Hey, I thought I was going to be a monkey when I grew up. *Really.* I remember hanging from thick tree branches and eating bananas and scratching under my arm, screeching as the monkey is known to do. I watched Tarzan faithfully every Saturday morning. I was set—until my dad broke the news that my intended life wasn't possible. That I would never be a monkey, because I was human, and humans don't have hairy bodies (okay some do!) and that I was not going to sit on tree limbs eating bananas and hang out with Tarzan and Jane.

I was devastated; my future was smashed—taken from me. I was three.

Sometimes we think we know what we're supposed to do, and that's not what we're supposed to do. I was hell-bent on becoming a stewardess when I was in high school and during my early years of college. I remained quite dedicated, to the point that I studied Spanish and French and starved myself for an interview only to be skipped over because I was five pounds above the requirement. I had lost over seventy-five pounds for the interview! Again, my dream of a glorious future was crushed. But perhaps that wasn't my intended bliss. Maybe we chase after something that's not meant to be, so instead we focus our life on the "off" time to be happy filling up with foods.

Perhaps the food fester's cheat day mentality is about covering up the fear of not having this bliss we are all so hungry for. You see our issue is not at all about the food—never was—never will be. It's about the empty we're so desperately trying to fill. In Nikko's case, he was suffering from a broken heart. He was missing the space Bruno had occupied, and would need time to heal. But he wasn't replacing his pain with drugs, alcohol, gambling, sex or food; no, he was feeling the feeling as gripping as it was.

Sometimes the Booze Calls

I recall Martha when her dog, Johnny, passed away. Within hours, she was combing the ads to replace him. She was honest with me in her therapy session, admitting she didn't want to *feel* this lonely, grinding ache in her heart. She wanted it gone as quickly as it had come on. Back in her drinking days, Martha covered her feelings with booze—now she embraced and owned her feelings, learning to pass through rather than around them.

But in this case, Martha didn't want to feel—nor did she want to drink. She chose to fill her empty with another furball. A few days later, she met Charley, and rescued him. Charley is a lovely dog, and for a minute he did fill the hole in her heart, but in time, Martha began drinking, an addiction she'd been in recovery from for years.

Thank goodness we caught it early, as we spoke of losses, digging deep into fears of abandonment and grief, stemming back to childhood, when she learned at the age of twelve that she was adopted. She felt empty, lost, and lied to. The sudden death of her dog reopened a wound she'd buried long ago. Once she began to understand what was eating away at her, she began recovery once again.

Martha learned you have to move through your feelings rather than skirt around them, because if you skip this important step, the grieving process is worse than you can ever imagine.

Perhaps you don't know how to feel your feelings, so you eat them, or like Martha, you drink them—or maybe drug them, or seek out some other way of masking your pain. Like Martha, if you mask what's really troubling you, it morphs into a fuzzy mess and may be buried with a substance such as food. But, in time, with self-analysis you learn the question isn't what you're eating, but rather what's eating you.

So when you endure the loss of a loved one, or you're off from work, and it's a long weekend, or an evening after a hard day at work, you may well give yourself over to goodies, drinks, or anything to fill the empty—or when it's your birthday and you're another year older, you fill with food.

You can see a pattern here. And this presents an opportunity, a chance to release your obsession with food festivities meant to fill the empty, and instead turn to looking into what it is that's eating you. Go deep, look internally, and what troubles you often will bubble up.

What Is Your Bliss?

I remember years back, I was soaking in the sun with my best friend, Yvonne, on our makeshift section of the beach, slathered in suntan lotion, listening to the sounds of the waves crashing on the shoreline and Dr. Dyer blaring from the boombox we'd toted along. Dr. Dyer has been an influencer in my life since my late teens when I'd read his first book, *Your Erroneous Zones.*

Yvonne was grabbing and sifting fistfuls of sand with one hand over and over in slow motion like an hourglass measuring time, gabbing about her dreams and aspirations, soaking in the sun, carefree. But at the same time, I was stressing about who I was and where I was going. *It's your thoughts that create these false beliefs* but how do you stop them when you don't know what to do?

At one point, Yvonne popped up, sand sticking to her oiled skin, reaching for the sky as if she were stretching toward the clouds while we listened to Dr. Wayne Dyer on a tape (this was the pre-digital age!) because she had that "ah ha" moment when she recognized she ***was*** living her bliss. Yvonne was good with staying in the now. She wasn't fixated on food, her body weight, or where she was going in her life.

We were on vacation and I was eating and eating and eating. I lay there on the sheet feeling as fat as a beached wale with no dreams, no goals, and nothing to look forward to—so I ate. Vacations are time to eat, right? I deserved it. Right? Heck what else are you supposed to do on vacation? I loved Florida; being on the beach felt good —felt like paradise.

On and on, we listened to Dr. Wayne Dyer with children splashing, running, and laughing, kicking up sand as they ran by. Unbeknownst to us we were naturally embarking on a pleasure trip—enjoying pure bliss while simply resting on the sheet, listening to crashing waves coming and going, with seagulls swooping down and children's laughter ringing out.

What's in Your Future?

Maybe what's eating you is the fear of not knowing where your future is going to take you. The point is not about finding your bliss, but rather accepting that maybe you don't know what your bliss is.

I was panic stricken that day on the beach because I intuitively understood this idea that something was eating me, rather than allowing my usual focus on what to eat. My inability to nail the nature of my bliss was my real problem. Bliss?

What the heck do I know about bliss? I thought.

I didn't really even get what bliss was. I was overthinking this concept. I recall Dr. Dyer making reference to some man who hated his job but lit up like a Christmas tree when he came home to play in his apple orchard. He loved making apple juice, applesauce, and apple pie. Dr. Dyer told him his bliss was his apple orchard…and the guy went on to become famous. I don't recall the name of the company that made his apple-based products, as this was over 35 years ago, but the company was quite successful and well known.

Today, my friend Yvonne is here no longer—she died only a few years after our beach excursion, ever-so-etched in my mind. She died in her bliss. She loved life and all that it offered. Her bliss was singing and psychology, and not exactly in that order. I then had no idea.

Yvonne liked to laugh and sing and enjoy herself with every morsel of her being, while I, self-conscious, pimple faced, overweight—lonely and frightened about what my next step would be in life even considered becoming a pest and bug exterminator! I know, I know...I was reaching. That you could earn money in a field you loved never occurred to me. At that time, I had no idea what I was going to do for a living.

We Don't Always Know—And It's Okay

I learned on that day I didn't have to know my bliss right that second. That my bliss was inside me, and it would be the *knowing* within which would bubble up at the right time without force. And it did…

Fast forward, my bliss today is writing and psychology. Yvonne died at 44 years old in her sleep. I believe she was blissfully happy for the most part. She danced to her own tune. She knew that she just wanted to be her authentic self. I loved that about her!

I learned a good deal about bliss watching Yvonne. She was one of my greatest teachers, as was Dr. Dyer, who also passed away—only a few years after he and his daughter Serena wrote: *Don't Die with Your Music Still in You.* How appropriate.

So what's really eating you? Is your concern the food or is it finding your authentic self? In Chapter 10, we'll consider the question while looking at the sad tale of Holiday Fog.

Personal Inventory Questions

1. What if the issue isn't actually what you eat and rather a matter of what's eating you? Could something be going on within that has nothing to do with food? Examine why you eat and you may be surprised at what you learn about yourself.
2. Dr. Dyer says the truth is that we have no actual stress or anxiety in the world; our thoughts create these false beliefs. Do you think Dr. Dyer is on to something? Do you think your beliefs (and fears) are created in your imagination?
3. Nikko's pain was real; he unexpectedly lost his best friend, Bruno, who traveled with him everywhere he went around the world. The two were inseparable. His grief wasn't about what he was eating, nor about what was eating him, but rather about real pain. Can you identify the difference

between what you're eating, what is eating you, and real pain that comes from a devastating situation?

4. I'm looking at this thing we do when we go into "vacation mode" and turn to food for fun, happiness, freedom, and whatever else we imagine this food fest frenzy will bring to us. Do you think the hoopla might be a cover for what's really going on?
5. Taking a close look at why we behave and think the way we do regarding food and vacation time, what have you learned about yourself?
6. Did you know what your bliss was as a child? What about now? How does this knowing or not knowing impact your free time as it relates to food fest frenzy?
7. Are you living your best life now? If not, what's missing and what would make your life more satisfying?
8. Two of the biggest influencers in my life were my best friend, Yvonne, and Dr. Wayne W. Dyer. Yvonne was one of my greatest teachers as was Dr. Dyer, both now passed. Do you have a mentor or a best friend who influenced your life? How did that person have an impact on you?
9. Dr. Dyer and his daughter Serena wrote: *Don't Die with Your Music Still in You.* How appropriate. What does this title bring up for you? What music do you still have in you?
10. What steps can you take to find your bliss?—whatever that might mean to you. You would do this something whether you were paid or not. Do you have something you love to do, but the time and that something slip by without you noticing it?

Chapter 10

Holiday Fog

Reality is merely an illusion,
albeit a very persistent one.
~Albert Einstein

Jingle, jingle, jingle all the way…cookies and candies, reindeer and glitter, a time to twirl, a time to whirl, a time to play, a time for magic. Chocolates and cookies, gumdrops and gingerbread, all swirling, and dancing in the head. No surprise, the illusion and reality, mixed and marred. It's holiday time: *a time to eat.*

Mom piled the gifts from the floor to ceiling for each of her six children to rip open early Christmas morning. Excitement rang throughout the house. Waiting, *tap, tap, tap*, waiting for Mom and Dad to wake up, so we could tear into the golden and red papers to learn our surprises. The house was quiet, nothing was stirring—not even a mouse.

As noted earlier, Dad was a well-known accordion player, and often played evenings at gala events for important people such as Richard Nixon. He opened for Liberace, and even turned down the opportunity to play the accordion as a regular on *The Lawrence Welk Show*—an American televised musical variety show hosted by big band leader Lawrence Welk.

So, sleeping-in was a must for Dad after he'd worked well into the late hours. To keep us children quiet, Mom lined us up along the wall in their bedroom to keep an eye on us. We sat Indian-style, *tap, tap, tap,* chomping at the bit to tear open our presents. Mischievous Michael inserted his finger in his nose, pretending to pick, or he lifted his rump as if to flatulate, and pulled faces—all of which started the six of us laughing—and got us in a heap of trouble.

Michael was a jokester, and still to this day presents some of the same pranks and silliness he displayed when we were little children. The memories are colored in a Brady Bunch kind of style that makes them more tolerable than the reality.

We often bump up memories to elaborate illusions, creating a joy that perhaps wasn't quite the reality. *Reality is merely an illusion, albeit a persistent one*, as Albert Einstein tells us.

We hold onto these exaggerated memories as if they're the truth, while often what happened isn't quite what we've created in our minds. The mind is a powerful tool that has a tendency to add and delete information that isn't always accurate. Why? Perhaps to muffle the reality that disappoints, thus enhancing the supposedly magical moment of holiday time.

Gobble, Gobble...

Though I certainly have delightful holiday memories, I also recall some not so good ones—like the time I had four of my molars extracted at nine years old. I had eaten so much candy they'd rotted down to the gums, causing excruciating pain every time I ate sweets or crunchy foods.

A few days before Thanksgiving, knees shaking, paralyzed in fear, I felt the dentist reach into my mouth and stuff it with what looked like an oversized square green eraser that smelled like a combination of rubber and airplane glue to prop open my mouth. He then hooked a mask over my face and told me to breathe in…*again*….*again*…*again*…while his face doubled, then tripled, and I drifted off, only to wake with my mouth stuffed with gauze.

Soon upon awaking, the pounding began—an unfamiliar ache substituting for the sharp toothaches that had become my norm. I was dazed and confused over what had just happened to me, which could explain my terror of dentists, not to mention my mother's own fear, which became mine. She always promised a treat of cookies or candy, or even a turtle one time as a bribe. Often the bribes never materialized—forgotten they were ever offered.

I then understood my neighbor's little nephew's fear when several of his teeth were extracted. They were taken out due to their rotting after he'd sucked on the baby bottle beyond the years he should have. I'd never dreamed such a thing could happen to me. But it surely did.

After my oral ordeal at the dentist's, once I was settled into my bed, I endured days of endless pain sipping on cool, sweet drinks and eating mashed foods. I was hungry, and our Thanksgiving celebration took place only days later. Imagine my agony sniffing the delicious smells of Thanksgiving wafting in the air—sweet potatoes, turkey, and stuffing, and such, while all I could consume were liquids and mashed foods.

I was so hungry for Thanksgiving foods that years and years later when I missed out on a Thanksgiving due to being alone and newly single with a toddler, I went to my boss's home to share *their* Thanksgiving, and once again grieved. As when I was a little kid, I missed out on *my* family traditions.

The only difference was that as an adult I could recreate the entire meal my mother would have made—which I did when I arrived back home that day. And the reality, once I began indulging, was not the imagined festivity.

Boo…Ghosts and Goblins, Oh MY

Strolling down the aisles of Wal-Mart or Sam's Club at the end of summertime, seeing Christmas decorations outshining Halloween and Thanksgiving decor is not uncommon these days. Why not? Let's get the hype out there and remind everyone the promise of sparkle and ecstasy soon to be upon us.

Side by side, ghost and goblin outfits, lit reindeer bobbing up and down, tins of cookies and candies, and everything bright, all folded into one big festivity blending Halloween and Christmas, all while outside it's blazing hot in my neighborhood, as summer still unwinds. This setup invites imaginings of what will be kids and out-of-control adults running wild, chasing the promise of rapture with cheat days folded in.

Holiday time is glamorized and commercialized to the hilt, making people feel that if they're not a part of these exciting times, they're missing out. And research shows depression is at its height during the weeks upon weeks of holiday time. I'm thinking the cause must be those darn Publix commercials (name your own grocery chain) showing the festivities with the perfectly groomed family—a table set as if for the queen of England, making us "regular" people feel less than…

This illusion opens up the mind-valve, imparting the message that the food and festivities are about to begin. The Cheat Day—Food Fest Frenzy in all its glory is knocking on the emotional door, saying, "Come on in…it's cozy inside—all the goodies of the season are here…and if you don't eat and partake, then you don't celebrate Hanukkah or Christmas, the two major religious holidays, celebrated by Jews and Christians in the United States, and of course, in places around the world.

With the holiday frenzy come houses lit with colorful lights, fancy wreaths on the doors, trees for some in their living rooms—all dolled up with glitter and gold and twinkle and bows. This is a time when we embrace family and friends—giving and attending holiday parties filled with sugar and spice and everything nice.

Family and religious traditions inspire many of these celebrations, but more and more the Yuletide has been commercialized into a buying and eating frenzy, completely missing the point of the celebration in the first place.

The goal of ***Release Your Obsession with Cheat DAZE: Heal from the Inside Out*** is for readers to break away from the belief that food is going to make us happy, regardless of the time of year or festivities in place. The message I want to send is that you don't have to be a Food Fester, gobbling up everything in sight, just in case you miss out.

Yes, food is a good thing—filled with nutrients, and definitely we should enjoy partaking in many of the holidays' delights. The problem is when the foods become our only focus and eating is out of our control to the point of misery, shame, and worse—continuing guilt. The problem is when we give in to the "treats" afforded by the standard American diet (remember SAD?), which consists of processed, unhealthy foods—often the primary offering during holiday time.

Perhaps we're missing the spiritual food that fills us with love and light. Perhaps the promise of gifts and holiday cheer is steering us from the assurance of a Higher Source's love, a gift that isn't costly and covered in glitter and gold, but natural and ever-present for ALL for the taking, regardless of color, nationality, riches or not.

This is not to say gathering with family is wrong, for certainly it is not—strength in loving numbers is a good thing as family gathers to connect. And food is a part of that gathering, which is also not wrong.

Food often is part of a celebration with others, including friends, co-workers, and family. We long for the association with others. We long for family connection, but somehow the idea and its reality have merged into the image of food fueling our happiness and food *becoming* the happiness. No, that's not what we want to do, because then we make the food our God—our everything, a step from the path, which only brings physical and spiritual ills and confusion.

The representation is that if you don't eat the "celebratory" foods, then you're missing out on the holiday season. Your merriment won't be quite on target with everyone else's. So you eat. And eat. And eat some more, until the food fog takes over, and you zombie walk your way through the holiday period, packing on weight, guilt, and the jitters that the food fog brings, starting with the handouts at ghost and goblin time.

That very Thanksgiving, I described above when I was single parenting my small son, who at the time was barely three years old, was quite telling about the illusions and fantasies we carry from childhood to adulthood. I didn't have family here in South Florida where I reside, so my Thanksgiving was to be spent alone. At the time, I worked for Weight Watchers of Greater Miami. The vice president got wind that I would be alone and invited me to her home to celebrate with her family. I'm quite shy but found saying no difficult, as the VP was a strong personality and ***no*** was not an option.

The event was full of glitter and gold, and everything delightful to eat. Did I say I was shy? Well, shy means you eat a meager amount because you feel awkward. When I returned home, I felt sad, as though I'd missed out on Thanksgiving, as I knew it at that time. I knew Thanksgiving as my stomach so stuffed I could barely move, and then after waiting a short while, repeating the process over and over a few more times…and then the leftovers… Yes, the leftovers.

I was searching for something that didn't exist. I wanted family and love, but I was alone with my toddler, while the rest of the world seemed to be partying and gathering. *The Publix commercials said so*, and they showed the lovely, decorated table, with fine china and glassware, and a well-groomed family, laughing and clinking glasses in a radiant atmosphere. The home of the VP ***so*** looked like a Publix commercial, but I was the odd woman out.

Thus, what did I do that year? I recreated Thanksgiving for two—me and a toddler who barely ate, but not to worry, I ate for me, I ate for him, and I ate for the entire world. Try as I might to create my remembered bliss, as I eventually learned, *the reality is merely an illusion, albeit a persistent one.* The past was gone and perhaps it never existed in the way I'd thought. Yes, Food Fest Frenzy…bring it on! I was conditioned to believe Thanksgiving to be a cheat day (or more than a day, considering the leftovers), as was Halloween, and of course Christmas too, winding down with New Year's Eve—and promising to do better in the coming year.

Holiday time doesn't have to be this way. Turn it around and make the celebration about family, friends, and God (or whatever Source you ascribe to)—and not necessarily in that order.

Perhaps you're not comfortable with the idea of God—then find your Source the way you understand it. Perhaps it's energy to you. Or, maybe your Source is found in nature, in the birds, in the trees, in the sky and the vast ocean that represents an infinite power to you. Fine. God is whatever God is to you.

And Then There Was Light

One holiday season I was working with a patient we'll call Markus, who was in a relationship with Matthew, a high-powered attorney, a man always out and about while Markus stayed in and minded the home. Markus studied medicine with the hope of becoming a doctor. But then tragedy struck. Markus had undetected acute bacterial meningitis, a rapidly developing inflammation of the layers of tissue that cover the brain and spinal cord (meninges) and of the fluid-filled space between the meninges (subarachnoid space) caused by bacteria.

Due to excess fluid putting pressure on the brain, the fluid needed to be drained. The condition is quite serious. People who have had meningitis may be subject to permanent mental impairment, problems with memory or concentration, learning disabilities, behavioral disorders, etc.

Markus was fortunate to catch the situation early and treat early, due to his medical background. He needed several operations and exhibited some of the symptoms described. At one point, he had a drain (shunt) placed in the brain to relieve increased pressure in the skull.

Markus became depressed and withdrawn and believed no such thing as God or any kind of supernatural energy existed whatsoever. The holiday came and went, as he buried himself in vats of food, making each day a cheat day, hoping to create something, *anything* so that he didn't have to feel. He signed up for the cheat day mentality, thinking this was the fix for all he endured. Not.

Matthew, unlike Markus, was light and loving, and full of energy and faith. He believed and he prayed. He saw joy in everything, and even during the tough times he found a way to see the good.

Then while under the surgical knife, only days before the holiday season was about to unfold, Markus had an experience. "He" rose above his body to look down and witness the surgeons working on his brain. He saw a light—a very bright light. He felt warm and safe. He felt loved.

Everything changed after that experience. He began to seek a God of his understanding. He wanted family, and embraced his friends. As Markus's healing became more and more apparent, this loving couple reached out to adopt a child, and eventually went on to adopt other children. Today, their home is filled with family—six kids to be exact. Markus healed to the point at which he returned to school and finished his education and now has a successful medical practice. Food no longer was his main attraction. He no longer experienced holiday brain fog. He treasured his brain, his thoughts, and his very life.

Let the Cheat Days Begin

Back in the day, my food fest frenzy under the influence of cheat day mentality began in a fury on Halloween and stretched all the way to New Year's Eve, when I made a promise to the universe that never ever again was I going to binge eat. And that vow lasted a good few hours into New Year's Day, and downhill I'd go, thinking after Valentine's Day—yes that was good. I'd start then…but of course Valentine's turned into waiting until Lenten season began.

For sure anyone would think a pact with God for my penance, from Ash Wednesday, with what seemed like an extra-large smudge of black ash on my forehead, I could quiet my obsession with food fest frenzy. Nope. I'd last a day or two, or maybe squeak in a week—but then that darn Cadbury bunny would come on, commercial after commercial, so who could wait for Easter to dig into the chocolate decadent egg with the creamy inside. And then they had to come up with dark chocolate—even more alluring.

Yes, it all began with Halloween…to New Year's to Valentine's, to Easter, and then, oh gosh, it's springtime, and summertime, and picnics, and oh my. A never-ending thrust of holidays coming and going, circling back to the jingle, jingle and holiday fog fury.

Memories of Once Was

When we were kids, we celebrated Halloween on the eve ***and*** on the actual day, so we had two days of dressing up as ghosts and goblins, filling our pillowcases with as much as we could carry, and then some.

I didn't care much for the dark scary creatures roaming the streets, but knowing I was accumulating candy made the venturing forth worth the while. At door after door, we gathered and collected. Mrs. Smith gave apples and Mr. Johnson raisins…those we tossed, along with the *"suspicious"* candies and baked goods that *could* have a razor blade hidden or some other lethal something. But did that stop me? Nope. Candy was my adrenaline—my drug before I even knew it was an addictive substance for me.

I mentioned in one of my books that I was the mother who stole my child's candy when he was fast asleep, his cowboy attire still in place, tuckered out after a night of trick or treating. We also sorted his pile of goods, and I'd say, "This doesn't look safe…oh, this one too…and oh look this wrapper is open some." And of course guess who was eating it later in the night while he was fast asleep.

The holiday fog isn't imagined or something that you caused—it's brought on by the wish that the goods will give you something that they can't—love, family, faith, friends.

When you release the obsession with cheat day mentality, you find recovery—you heal from the inside out. You discover connections with *Source* far richer and deeper than any sugary, starchy concoction can give you –even though the promise is that the food will make your holiday magical as the magazines filling up the racks in the grocery store suggest. *It's an illusion.* The truth is the friends, family, and your Higher Source are going to fill you with what you're looking for—now that's reality.

And the story doesn't end there because sugar, fat, and salt (Chapter 11) is enticing us toward every food from sweet to sour, crunchy to creamy—conditioning and tempting us with processed foods at every turn.

Personal Inventory Questions

1. Do you think reality is merely an illusion, albeit a persistent one? What reality nags at you? How do you decipher what is real and what is an illusion?
2. In what ways are your holiday seasons filled with glitter and spice, everything nice?
3. What parts of the eating patterns described in this chapter resonate with you? When did you first notice you couldn't stop after just one cookie or potato chip, or whatever your addictive food was/is?
4. Do you try and recreate your childhood holidays? Were they magical or difficult? Is your creation an illusion of what you thought it was—or what you wished it could be?
5. Do you have memories of eating and eating, and eating some more during the Thanksgiving weekend? Was that the start of your holiday fog? Or did you begin at another holiday season?
6. What role did Halloween play in your eating frenzy? Do you have childhood memories of running up and down the streets, sweating in your costume, collecting all the goodies you could possibly carry? Or perhaps your family didn't allow a celebration with the witches and dragons, and you felt left out? What is your memory and how has it impacted you?
7. Do you create for your children, family, or friends the same holiday season you grew up with, or did you carve out your own personal style that represents the jingle that's about to unfold?
8. What would the season be like for you if you made peace, love, and your connection to the God of your understanding the top priority in your holiday bash? And if you already do, as surely some of you do, what got you to that place? Was that the norm or is that now the norm?

9. Did you ever have an operation like Markus or perhaps like me, or some type of a medical condition during the holiday season that impacted you? How does it manifest for you?
10. Can you imagine making your family and friends the priority during the season? Would that change the way you look at festivities without cheat day mentality going forward?

Chapter 11

Sugar, Salt, Fat

Then God said, "I give you every seed-bearing plant on the face of the whole earth and every tree that has fruit with seed in it. They will be yours for food."
~Genesis 1:29

Yikes. Okay, what does the quote from Genesis mean? If every food is available to me, then bring it on. Yes, to fat, sugar, and salt—the three most addictive foods. No, wait a darn minute, these are the addictive foods, right? Yes, indeed they are. Well then, why were they provided for me to eat if they're not good for me?

If you're not a food addict, as described in Chapter 12, then yes, bring it on. If you're not struggling with your moods and attention span, yes, bring it on. If you're of a good weight for your height, age, and build, certainly ***bring it on***. Eat away, in moderation of course.

But if you're suffering from the inability to stop eating, and your weight is beginning to soar, and you feel simply awful, then you might want to reconsider these foods, especially given a road trip where processed high-fat, salty, and sugary foods are served in nearly every restaurant, truck stop, and drive-through in the nation.

You see, when you're in vacation mode, and birthday mode, and oh yes, it's-the-weekend mode, then you'll run into an overabundance of sugar, processed fat, and salt. Restaurants lavish these three ingredients on diners in most of their foods, as do the majority of packaged food makers, and certainly the fast food enterprises. Yes, these are foods that will keep you eating, and wanting, and feeling awful.

So yes, God said, "I give you every seed-bearing plant on the face of the whole earth and every fruit that has seed in it. They will be yours for food to eat."

What to do? Well, let's go back to the basics. Eat the foods that are from the earth, from the sea, from the sky, and from the tree—*in their natural forms.* The goal is to clear out your palate. When you eat sugar, you want more sugar. When you eat salt, guess what—you want more salt. And yep, when you eat processed fat, you want more fat. For this reason, eating high-sodium foods and high-fat foods is dangerous, not to mention, foods laced with sugar. And the high-carb diet is not a good deal, either. Nor is the high-protein diet.

The key is balance. ***B…A…L…A…N…C…E….***

Move away from the sugary, salty, high-fat processed foods, and into foods from the earth, eaten at regular intervals, with a wide variety of God's earthly foods, and you are headed in the right direction.

Mickey Mouse Here We Come

Yvonna, a bubbly Italian-American woman in her early thirties with voluptuous curves, loves food and celebration. She has an infectious laugh, and for sure she's the life of the party. Family gatherings are extremely important to her.

At one time, after the birth of her son, followed by a daughter, Yvonna carried thirty pounds more than she felt comfortable lugging around. She wanted to release the weight, but didn't want to let go of her "traditional" rituals, which she was quite attached to.

You see, Yvonna couldn't imagine going to Disney World, her favorite go-to place *in the world,* without eating Twizzlers' red braided licorice sticks, salty/vinegary chips, and Hershey's Kisses. That's what she'd eaten as a kid, and she expected to do the same forevermore as they rolled down the highway toward Mickey Mouse.

Yvonna associated love, family, and vacation as being all wrapped alongside red licorice and vinegar chips, doused with a finale of Hershey's Kisses melting on her tongue with blissful happiness.

You say, "What's wrong with that!??" Why can't Yvonna embrace blissful happiness with her edible delights? Well, first because Yvonna can't stop the indulgence at that, and second, because the 'treats" make her anxious, irritable, and very, very depressed after she bounces from her sugar high to a deflated low.

The truth of the matter is that Yvonna is really NOT happy or in bliss, but rather feeling lonely, even with a car full of family, noise, music blaring in the background, and wind blowing in her face—as often the windows are open to let in the warmth of the Florida sun. The sweet-smelling breeze whips across her face flipping her long, wavy auburn hair this way and that.

All this echoes early childhood days that she tries to recreate with her family of now. Her imagination created a trip full of love, and promise, and joy. Yes, for sure the family of origin was a loving family, but also was a family in turmoil. Dad fought with Mom, who fought with Grandma, who fought with Grandpa, while Stepmom felt left out, and Stepdad was disconnected from the whole scene. Mom's mom and dad were permissive and giving.

Yes, happy and sad, all rolled into one memory of licorice, chips, and melting chocolate.

Yvonna, prone to panic attacks and anxiety since a road trip after the birth of her daughter, now fears going away whether in a car or plane, or even a train—expecting an episode. On that particular trip when she was a new mother, her now family was headed on a road trip to Canada. Unexpectedly, her heart began to pound out of her chest, while sweat beaded up on her forehead, and she had to get out of the car, fearing impending doom. *Nothing had happened to bring this on.*

Everyone was singing to the radio, passing the treats back and forth, swigging down sweetened soda pops. Everything was good—until it wasn't.

All of a sudden, out of nowhere, all color washed from Yvonna's face, and she began to tremble uncontrollably. She screamed, "Stop the car. I have to get out. NOW!" She was dying, having a heart attack, perhaps. She couldn't breathe. Her world was cascading inward as her family's voices became muffled. Winglets of hair stuck to her cheeks, and sweat poured out of her.

Mike, her husband and best friend, called 911. Shortly after, the paramedics arrived. Off to the ER, Yvonna went. A few hours later, she was discharged, anti-anxiety meds in hand, completely disheartened that she'd ruined the trip. They went home rather than to Canada. Yvonna had experienced a full-blown panic attack.

Soon after the incident, Yvonna made her first psychotherapy appointment with me. We explored her life history and uncovered a loud, chaotic, yet loving childhood, with four sets of grandparents, and two sets of parents, as Dad remarried, and so did Mom. Yvonna was an only child at the time, and none of her parents' siblings had children. She was it.

All the attention went to Yvonna. One of the grandmas picked her up from school daily, taking her to the local donut shop for a soda and donut, while the other grandma made cookies and pies with her every weekend. The other two sets of grandparents when in town popped in and out of her life with lovely brownies, chocolate kisses, and the like.

The two sets of parents worked and were on budgets, so they turned to fast food and junk food as the daily staple. With the two close sets of grandparents and the two sets of parents, not to mention the other two sets of grandparents who randomly appeared, Yvonna received plenty of attention—*and plenty of sugar, salt, and processed fat.*

One of the places Yvonna most adored was Disney World, which became her go-to refuge just about every other month. Disney, a make-believe world, promised all the magic and safety a little girl could imagine.

Every year, Yvonna went to Disney with each set of parents, then grandparents—making it an event every couple of months. And yes, sugar, fat, and salt—bring it on!!

The ride to the Magic Kingdom was filled with music and treats to devour. Yvonna loved to take the licorice braids apart with her teeth, making several little skinny strings to eat, and tying one around her finger, crafting a pretend ring that every princess needs, matching the crown she wore along with her pink dress. While on the amusement park grounds, she demolished French fried potatoes, sugar cones, and cotton candy, not to mention bags and bags of various assorted sweets.

This was love to Yvonna—sugar, salt, and fat—*and everything nice.* These delivered attention, love, and whatever was yummy. The world felt right—the world felt safe. So how on earth could she not do the same for her own children? But the doctors warned her that this wasn't helping her blood pressure, not to mention her anxiety. She was told to see a doctor for her nerves. And so she did.

Yvonna didn't have a health issue per se, but rather she had hypoglycemia that caused the lows, then ate sugar, flour, and salt that brought on the highs. Hypoglycemia refers to low levels of sugar (glucose) in the blood. It, in itself, is not a disease, but it can indicate a serious health problem. All the body's cells, including the brain, need energy to function. In Yvonna's case, she was depleting her brain and body's cells of good nutrition. Signs of low blood sugar include: hunger, trembling, heart racing, nausea, and sweating.

Yvonna was not a diabetic, but she was at risk to becoming diabetic, given her family's history. Yvonna preferred to eat sugary foods along with high-fat processed foods, and loved her salt. She barely ate a meal with actual nutrition. Her staples consisted of French fried potatoes plus chicken nuggets from the Golden Arches, a meal topped off with a chocolate shake. This was an almost daily ritual. The other meals—if you could call them that—were candy, chips, licorice, and tons of soda pop—root beer to be exact.

Yvonna learned she needed to change her diet by eating small meals and snacks throughout the day. The best treatment for her was to eat real food every three hours. She was advised to have a variety of foods, including protein, fatty foods (good fats of course!), and high-fiber foods, such as fruit, oatmeal, and vegetables. Yvonna's doctor suggested a high-protein, low-carbohydrate diet, given her hypoglycemia alongside her food addiction, not to mention her panic attacks that had evolved after "the" trip to Canada, or as Yvonna would say, "The trip to hell and back."

Yvonna made a complete turnaround. She changed her lifestyle by getting up each morning without fail an hour-and-a-half before the rest of the family stirred, so she could drink a hot tea and write in her journal, followed by a period of meditation, and then exercise. After giving self-love, she was ready for a delicious, nutritious, engaging breakfast with her children. This was huge for the family, as normally she stopped at Dunkin' Donuts on the way to their schools, snagging donuts and chocolate milk for the two.

At first the kids weren't happy with this "healthy" swap of foods. No longer did they stop on the way to their schools, and instead Mom cooked at home. This was huge! She began with a breakfast of real foods to start her day right and nourish the kids. Soon her blood levels began to normalize, and she for once *wanted* fruits and vegetables, good sources of protein, and healthy starches. She felt fabulous. Slowly and steadily, her weight returned to what was right for her.

What's My Brain Got to Do with It?

Food addiction has gotten a bum rap these days. Now instead of calling it as it is, the name is "sugar coated" (no pun intended) and labeled an eating addiction. I suppose we can think of the familiar vegetable (fruit) as tomato *(tomayto)* or tomato *(tomahto)*, depending on where you're from, but at the end of the day, it's still a tomato. At the end of the eating addiction tag, you'll find a food addiction, and vice versa.

And while we're on the subject of food addiction, or brain addiction, we need to look at compulsive eating, which only confuses the matter more. Compulsive eating, from my perspective as an eating disorder specialist and food addict in recovery, is really not any different than compulsive drinking or smoking. The same chemical imbalance drives all three.

Like Yvonna, perhaps you learned as a child to eat to feel better, and the foods that helped you feel best (at least for the moment of consumption) were probably high in fat and/or cooked with enriched white flour, and full of sugar, like donuts, cookies, ice cream, French fries, and potato chips. This is known as the palatable food problem because it lights up the same addictive dopaminergic pathway as cocaine, ensuring that once you start with that substance, you'll crave more!

While waiting for this brain signal, Yvonna couldn't stop eating. Low serotonin levels initiate carbohydrate cravings, and are also responsible for the brain not knowing how to detect in a timely manner that the stomach is full—that is before too much food is consumed.

As noted with Yvonna, who picked up 30 pounds eating without knowing she was full, it's the kind and quantity of food that causes weight gain. Fresh fruits and vegetables with lean proteins, good sources of rich high-fiber starchy carbs, and quality fats such as virgin olive oil and coconut oil aren't the culprits. The simple carbohydrates, such as sweets, and foods made from refined sugars and flours are what have the chemical structure that can be more readily stored as fats in the body, especially if they're eaten in quantities that aren't burned off as energy.

This is not to say that carbohydrates are the bad guys, as some seem to tout these days, and to make matters worse, too many people with low serotonin opt for no-carb diets that can magnify weight problems long term. You see, when they stop eating the carbs, they stop medicating the low serotonin feeling, and start to feel bad—really bad. And of course, soon they become too uncomfortable physically and emotionally, and guess what they do? Yep, they turn to the processed carbs. So, all you high-protein dieters out there, think again…you're creating a perfect storm…particularly for those of you who are food addicts.

Complex carbohydrates, which are whole, unprocessed foods containing naturally occurring vitamins, minerals, and fiber, require the body to work harder (burn more calories) in their digestion, and are a longer-lasting fuel source than simple carbohydrates. So, if you think you tend to gain weight when eating carbohydrates, take a closer look. Perhaps you're eating processed carbs, which is no different than eating a nice slice of cardboard. Yum.

Choose complex carbohydrates such as non-starchy vegetables and berries, in combination with your quality proteins, fat, and dairy, and you'll not only burn through them, you'll actually feel better because eating an adequate amount of complex carbohydrates throughout the day is an important element in the amino acid conversion process that leads to balanced brain chemistry.

Balance is the key here. A person with low serotonin levels eating high protein and saying no to extremely low carbohydrates is feeding the brain a poor quality fuel that spikes energy, but also robs the brain of serotonin by eating competing chemicals, and shortchanges the brain by not eating a sufficient amount of complex carbs to help the right chemicals cross the blood-brain barrier.

The long-term effect is that serotonin levels can be lowered even further, increasing depression, along with a felt need to engage in all the behaviors that promote weight gain in order to feel better.

A quick 101 lesson in food addiction, binge eating disorder, and compulsive eating: Food addiction is a disease that is characterized by a loss of control over the ability to stop eating certain foods. Furthermore, a person can become addicted to the chemical reactions resulting from the consumption of particular foods. Guess which foods these might be? Yep, fat, sugar, and salt.

A chemical dependency on food can be likened to the dependency of a drug user who becomes addicted to the high or euphoria experienced when abusing their substance of choice. I cover this subject extensively in my first of the Release Your Obsession Series, a book about food addiction: *Release Your Obsession with Food: Heal from the Inside Out.*

Binge eating is quite similar to food addiction, as the food addict always binge eats. The difference is that the binge eater is not always a food addict. The binge eater, like the food addict, eats a large amount of food, but not with the same gripping, chemical dependency you find in the food addict. The binge eater's addiction is more of a behavioral type rather than physiological. A compulsive eater manifests as virtually the same as a binge eater and may not be addicted, but again the food addict always is a compulsive eater.

Recovery Takes Hold

The other day Yvonna came in for a session and began to describe a lovely trip she made to Disney, a tradition she kept for her children—but now sans the Hershey's Kisses, salty vinegar chips, and red licorice for the long ride. Instead, she brought grapes, apples, and blueberries, along with slices of carrots, peppers, and cucumbers, and lemonade sweetened with fruits. Everyone sang and laughed the entire trip.

And Yvonna smiled from ear to ear, because she was able to keep her "me time," by getting up earlier than the kids to sip on her tea, write in her journal, meditate, and exercise. It never ever, *ever* occurred to her prior to the trip that she could incorporate this type of lifestyle on a jaunt to Disney and feel great, with not an inch of a sense of deprivation.

This can happen to you too. You can go to your weekend getaway and not have to lean on sugar, fat, and salt and really not miss these at all. When you stay away from these foods, you don't want them, and if too much fat, salt, or sugar is put in your food by accident, your food isn't palatable because it's too salty or too greasy or too sweet.

Food addiction, as I speak of in Chapter 12, can play a huge role in your cravings, moods, and overall poor health as you will soon learn.

Personal Inventory Questions

1. Do you make excuses why you need to eat this or that during a road trip? Where does this stem from? Pinpoint times in your childhood and compare those to your adulthood. Perhaps you're continuing and passing down this pattern to your children.
2. What are your go-to foods when you travel? Make a list of your foods that are whole, natural, healthy foods, and which tend to be processed. Trace back to where you began this habit (question 1) so you can slowly begin the process of switching to better-quality foods.
3. Are you attached to a memory of some sort, or do you associate travel with that specific food? So now that you have a list of foods, take a step back and analyze the memories attached to these. Are you more invested in the memory than the food?
4. What happens to you physically when you don't eat nutritious foods? Often we feel irritable, sluggish, *hangry* (a combination of hunger and anger) within an hour or so of eating. Make a list of how you feel.
5. Are you struggling with moving into a self-love ritual? In life we are taught to assist others but rarely taught to love and nurture ourselves—we're told that it's self-indulgent and selfish. What can you do for you that would show self-love, and self-care?
6. What are your thoughts as you read through the trials and tribulations of Yvonna? Can you relate? Make your own personal story of trials and tribulations, and then map your way to triumphs as Yvonna learned to do through her challenges.
7. Do you have family commotions with your current family, and/or family of origin? How can you create an atmosphere more conducive to peace and tranquility—a Zen space so to speak?

8. What's the one takeaway from this chapter that you can implement in your own healthy lifestyle? Begin to work this into your life a little at a time and soon it will become your new norm.
9. Do you worry your family will be upset if you switch to healthful foods as opposed to fast foods and processed foods? I so get that—as I was a bit concerned, too. But now, all these years later, I look back and realize I started a new trend for the generations to follow—imagine that you can as well.
10. What are your plans to improve your lifestyle? Make a chart of pros and cons from where you are to where you want to be. Get creative—perhaps make a vision board from magazine cutouts to create your dream life.

Chapter 12

Food Addiction

Above all else, guard your heart,
for everything you do flows from it.
~Proverbs 423

The food fester laced in cheat day mentality is not always a food addict but can simply be a foody caught up in eating for entertainment rather than out of hunger, and not due to needing nutritional supplies to sustain life. Eating is *a thing to do.* Yet while for most people eating is not all about the food, for the food addict it is.

Food addiction is real, and it is gripping. For food addicts, every thought, every behavior, every minute is about acquiring food, wherever they go, whatever they do, and whoever they're with. For some, food can be as addictive as cocaine or alcohol—or any addictive substance for that matter.

You might be thinking that's ridiculous. How can food be addictive? We have to eat to sustain life. Yes, we do have to eat to sustain life. And for most, food addiction isn't an issue, just as alcohol, or even marijuana for those who partake, isn't an issue—but for some it surely is. And you might be that someone as I was.

Moreover, if you're addictively eating, you most likely are suffering. *Above all else, guard your heart, for everything you do flows from it.* So, we definitely want to touch on the subject, because wherever you go, the food addict in you follows. Meet this head on, and squashing the binger in you can be accomplished—so that as a result, you can freely go wherever you wish and work your healthy eating. But first, let's take a peek at what food addiction is and how to move through it.

You Can Stop Thinking About Food

This book is written for those who can't stop thinking about food and who use holidays, weekends, parties, and any event, including funerals, to partake in overindulgences of food with cheat-day entitlement.

This book is to show you the way out of the "gotta eat" because I'm off from my everyday responsibility mentality. We don't have to eat junk food or be out of control with our foods. And even if you don't have any eating disorder or food addiction, do you really want to put processed foods into your body?

So, how do you stop? The first step is to remove the foods that cause you to eat out of control in the first place. Most often those foods include sugar, flour, and wheat. I know you're saying "but everything has those ingredients in it." No, not necessarily. True, many foods do contain these components, because they're addictive and purposely put in foods in the first place to keep you eating them. But you have plenty, and I mean plenty, of healthful, real foods to choose from that will wake up your taste buds and put a smile on your face.

Yes, sugar, flour, and wheat are in many foods—even items that you'd never, ever imagine have sugar in them.

Did you know cigarette manufacturers put sugar in their tobacco products? Yep, sugar. Why? So you keep smoking them. Yes, of course the tobacco is addictive too, but put a little sugar in there, and you sweeten the fix.

And what about potato chips? Why on earth do they put sugar in potato chips? Why? Sugar is in the chip because this addictive substance makes the chips more desirable, tapping at your subconscious that you want another—and another—and still another. That's why the commercial says, "You can't eat just one." They know darn well what they're making, and how to assure that you *need* it.

I recall a course I taught on health and nutrition in which healthy eating and lifestyle was the main focus. I had to laugh the first day when students inevitably walked into the classroom with their "healthy" foods: pretzels, sugar-free diet sodas, granola bars, and whatever food is generally advertised as being *good for you*, though it's in fact processed.

Tampered Foods

One day in my healthy eating class in particular is etched in my mind. We watched a documentary on corporations and how they put together foods for marketing. This requires an entire team: marketers, business-side persons, organizational psychologists, scientists, and a host of others sitting around a conference table, discussing how they can make the food so good the consumer *has* to have it. And these are the very foods that are addictive.

One psychologist was hired to look at consumers' emotional attachment to a product and the addictive components. And scientists worked on the physical need for more, while the engineers were packaging, and promotion was accomplished by marketing items that looked so good you could lick the wrapper. Are you shocked? I was. I had no idea that these people sit at tables thinking up ways to get their hooks into YOU to want the product, to dream and jones for it—and to not be able to stop at one.

Not only are companies sitting around plotting how to make the foods taste, look, and smell good, they're working at endlessly marketing to attract your attention. Sure, these companies always marketed, but the Berkeley Media Studies Group, in an article entitled "The New Age of Food Marketing: How Companies are Targeting and Luring Our Kids—and What Advocates Can Do About It" notes that the explosion of digital culture in recent years has dramatically changed the playing field and the rules, especially for children and teenagers, and companies marketing fast food, snack food, and soft drinks are at the forefront of the game.

Further, to make matters worse, marketers are tracking teens online and by cell phone, mining conversations on Facebook and Twitter, collecting data to develop and record personalized behavioral profiles.

And this is happening to adults too. When I was researching the ketogenic diet, to better understand what all the fuss was about, I began to notice keto advertisements everywhere. Since then, keto pops up on all the social media channels I hang out on. And I'm getting emails, including from Amazon, inquiring if I want to purchase products, food, and books, relating to keto.

Imagine all the places you hang out on your phone and computer are acquiring little trackers, knowing what you're interested in, and reminding you when you forget. So imagine further, you suffer from food addiction, or binge eating disorder, or a combination of the two, making you a sitting target, with all the gooey, sugary, and fried foods out there.

When I first began recovery, I was only dealing with the television commercials trying to tempt me in. At that period we had recorders with VHS—videotapes—to capture a favorite show, and for the first time we could watch when we wanted to, not when it aired—and more importantly, we could fast forward and move past all those persuasive commercials. That feature saved me from my own self and the outings that once happened *after* watching a commercial. But times have changed both for the better and for the not so great where foods are concerned.

In fact, in its report the Berkeley Media Studies Group notes that today one in three teens is either overweight or obese, and that overweight young people are likely to stay overweight throughout their lives. This puts these young people at risk for serious health issues going forward. And very likely many will be addicted to these specific, addictive foods throughout their lives.

But that said, many foods are clean and whole, taste fantastic, and quiet the fanatical need to eat junk foods. Eat, I say eat. But eat what is whole and clean and feeding your brain. Stay away from the foods that you can't get out of your head, as those most likely are the ones you're addicted to.

Did you ever notice you feel wonderful after certain meals, and not so good after others? Did you ever notice your mood starts to go south—you become irritable and moody—after a sugar high? This is food sensitivity. Maybe you aren't a food addict, but you are diabetic, or hypoglycemic, or maybe you have gluten sensitivity.

Death by Gluten

I read and reviewed Riya Anne Polcastro's book *Death by Gluten: How Undiagnosed Celiac Almost Cost Me My Life* and was amazed to see many of her challenges were similar to mine. If I didn't know better, I would have guessed she had food addiction, as many of the signs were there. She was irritable and moody, had trouble concentrating, and was fatigued most of the time, without knowing why. She just wanted to have fun and eat what she wanted.

Riya didn't have a weight issue; she had a food issue. Maybe you too have a food issue, not a weight issue—but in either case the solution is about respecting your body, which is sacred, so that you can heal on the inside, and the outside.

Why is this important to you, someone who simply wants a weekend off, or a birthday celebration, or a trip to Europe? Maybe you're thinking, *Why can't I just have fun—this is not fun.* Ah, here lies part of the problem. Why are we building our fun around food, rather than love? *Above all else, guard your heart, for everything you do flows from it.*

Everything you do is about life and love—not food. Yes, I know, I know food sustains our life. Yes, it does. But food doesn't have to be dripping in goo to make you happy. It doesn't have to possess that kind of hold on you.

Are You a Night Eater?

Betty, a flamboyant redhead, came barreling down the hallway heading toward my office, chatting. "Dr. Lisa, I did it again. I woke up in the middle of the night and binge-ate cereal!" As we made our way to my office, people in the waiting room and around the reception area raised their heads to see what the commotion was about.

When Betty arrived, all knew.

Betty was a spunky, loud woman, closing in on 70 years of age, with the most contagious laugh. Just thinking about Betty as I write this makes me smile from ear to ear. Betty is a handful—but also a total delight. She is unique, and eccentric, and most of all fun.

Betty started night eating several years back, after her father became quite ill. Nighttime eating has been linked to some eating disorders, including binge eating disorder, and night eating syndrome. People with night eating syndrome present a delayed food intake pattern, eating most of their dietary intake between late evening and early morning. Night eating syndrome is an eating disorder, characterized by a delayed circadian pattern of food intake.

Night eating syndrome differs from binge eating in that the amount of food consumed in the evening, or late night, is usually not a large amount of food, nor is it a loss of control over food intake required.

Betty left behind the comforts of her own home and moved in to care for dad as he declined. On many nights, in a blind-stupor, Betty consoled herself with a bowl of cereal, which turned into consuming the entire box.

Betty has binge-eating disorder *and* food addiction, and spent many years in and out of various twelve-step programs. She also sought a wide variety of therapists before she happened on me. I knew what she was going through as more than 20 years before, I binge ate and suffered from food addiction for quite some time until I found the resolution.

I invested years of education, first with my Master's degree in mental health, followed by a PhD in addictions with the emphasis on food addiction—and from there I obtained a certification in addictions, a Master's as a certified addiction professional (MCAP) and a certification in eating disorders as a certified eating disorder specialist (CEDS).

And then to top it off, I wrote two prior books on the subject: *Release Your Obsession with Food: Heal from the Inside Out* and *Release Your Obsession with Diet Chatter: Heal from the Inside Out*—and now a third book, *Release Your Obsession with Cheat DAZE: Heal from the Inside Out.*

I thought I was the only one who practiced as a clinician, as an expert in the field of eating disorders, and had personally worked through my own eating disorder, until I read a most interesting article in *Psychology Today*: "How to Stop Binge Eating in Three Unusual Steps" written by Glenn Livingston, Ph.D.

I was astounded and thrilled to learn about someone who mirrored much of what I have written and practiced over the past twenty-five years. Reading from his perspective was refreshing and enlightening.

I love the line in Dr. Livingston's article where he says, "I'll spare you the full story, but let's just say there's probably nothing you've done with food I haven't done myself." Oh my. I found my twin from another mother. He gets it! His riveting article goes on to point out three steps to overcome binge eating that ring similar to my perspective on many levels, yet are unique to his formula.

Dr. Livingston came to the same conclusions I did with Betty in regard to night eating. Betty for sure wasn't eating enough during the day and was making up for it big-time in the evening. Of course her eating pattern had emotional components with the decline of her father, but so too did the fact she was eating high, sugary foods in the late morning, followed by long periods of no food, after which she had a quick fast-food pick-me-up, and then went off to bed without proper nutrition, and without having eaten at regular intervals.

I concur with Dr. Livingston that treating and calling a halt to binge eating doesn't have to be difficult. He states, "Identifying the cause is a good starting place." He points out that over-restricting during the day—which was exactly what Betty was doing—along with not enough self-care during the day—which was absolutely part of Betty's pattern of self-denial—when reversed is also a remedy for binge eating.

Betty was too busy caring for her father and neglecting the care of herself…except during the night, when she'd overeat. Dr. Livingston also comments on the problem of not enough sleep, which is an area Betty and I, too, worked on. I emphasized the importance of good sleep at the same time each evening, if she could, and waking at the same time to create a blueprint, or a ritual that becomes a norm.

Dr. Livingston and I part ways with reference to how we treat binge eating disorder. I come from a place of love, teaching patients to love themselves, where Dr. Livingston, in his book *Never Binge Again: Reprogram Yourself to Think Like a Permanently Thin Person* focuses on mastering rules and discipline. This, he states, is how we increase freedom, by referencing your Pig self. Yes, you read that right—your Pig self.

Dr. Livingston's Pig self-analogy, reminds me of on Oprah's OWN when she had a series at a treatment center for eating disorder. I recall how one fellow who didn't do something right had to wear a paper bib held by a rope around his neck. On the paper was a picture of a pig. No, that's not self-care and self-love, that's belittling the self, with a militant approach, which the food addict and binge eater already do plenty of.

Though Betty is not quite out of the woods with her nighttime eating, the problem has ameliorated considerably in respect to the amount of food and the regularity of the event. She has gone from nightly eating seven times a week to falling into the practice two evenings every other week. She has learned to prepare healthy meals throughout the day and spaces them apart, and has to the best of her ability moved away from sugar, flour, and wheat, which ignite chemicals in her brain, fueling her food addiction.

Binge eating disorder can be a tough disorder to beat, or it can be an easy fix with the right tools.

The Long Weekend

Recently, my Easter weekend turned into a long festivity from Thursday thru Monday with food, kayaking, building a fireplace, and walking along the beach while in prayer.

My family took advantage of the break, escaping to my getaway to get away.

My getaway is a place where I suffered through many, many eating-frenzy moments in my youth. Easter, particularly, was a time to eat and be carried away with the previously mentioned Cadbury Creme Egg filled with a luscious soft center. I was an active, full-blown food addict, eating large amounts of food in a short period of time more days than not—until I'd hit a scary high weight, and then would start to diet, only to repeat the process. A vicious cycle indeed.

Times have changed. I no longer need to escape with food in the forefront. This trip, we shared many delectable meals, all clean and all filling. I experienced no jonsing, as I once had. Why? I'm in recovery. I don't eat sugar, flour, or wheat. Simple, yes. Profound, without a doubt.

Now, rather than pure indulgence in foods, which caused a huge disruption in my life, I guard my heart, because everything does flow from it. Life and recovery are about family and embracing the moment. They aren't about the food. And this Easter weekend was no different. No chocolate bunnies, Cadbury Creme Eggs, or squishy marshmallow chicks were to be found. And nobody missed them, or inquired.

Out on the fresh seas, paddling, going nowhere particular, with Pandora, Benjamin's boxer, at the helm, we made our way to the sandbar—what looked like a mini island to me. Pandora leaped out of the kayak, exploring, splashing, and running every which way. She was so happy, so free.

Once we landed securely on the sand, I got out to explore as well. Moving along in the squishy sand, delighted to find shells along the way, I happened upon a conch, and proudly carried it around. The more I walked, the squishier the sand became, and sinking to my ankles, glancing down to my now hidden feet, I saw glistening bluish bubbles—JELLY FISH!!

I screamed and began to try and make my way back to the boat, Benjamin behind me laughing at my squeamishness and my escape from brave exploring. My feet plunged deep into the sticky sand substance, feeling that they were being sucked down beneath the goo, with each attempt to lift out a struggle—desperate to return to my kayak.

Almost to the kayak, I became distracted by something blackish near my hand. A long, black, hairy leg was making its way out of the conch, wiggling toward contact with my skin. Screaming, and flailing my arms, I dropped the conch and trudged as quickly as I could back to the boat, eager to depart the little island.

Okay, so I'm not ever going to be a jungle explorer wandering through undiscovered nature. The city girl in me never left. Back to the makeshift fireplace, writing my stories is best for me. Oliver, my Eclectus parrot, and Southern Grace, my white Swiss shepherd, will have to do to keep the paradise feeling going.

We sat on the swing, on the dock, and around the fireplace—shared succulent burgers stuffed with onions, roasted Brussels sprouts, and baked potatoes for one evening meal, and had lovely breakfast banana pancakes for another repast. We laughed, and prayed, but never did we engage in eating processed foods.

Okay, hold the fort, that's not quite true. My son and his wife did go out for ice cream and enjoyed a beautiful block of chocolate, compliments of Swiss Chalet Fine Foods, where I'd given a talk only weeks before. But my son and his wife don't have an eating disorder, a fixation on food, or the inability to stop. So, for them, an occasional indulgence is just fine.

Paulina Arrests Binge Eating

Paulina, a lovely blonde, bronze skinned, blue-eyed Latina girl, came to see me about her inability to stop eating. She first had the lap-band surgery, but found the carbs she was sneaking caused her to throw up, and soon she became bulimic. She wanted to eat her bread and be skinny too. Sound familiar? In time, her stomach began to twist, and she was headed for some serious trouble.

Paulina begged and pleaded with the doctor to not remove her band. She was terrified she'd gain back her weight. But remove it he did. And yes, she began to gain back her weight, in between bouts of throwing up her food. She then went for the gastric sleeve—which doesn't indicate full, as the band did.

Paulina soon learned no surgery is going to remove food addiction. Just in case you missed this: *No surgery is going to remove food addiction.* And guess what? No drug is going to remove it either.

"But what if I have binge eating disorder?" Paulina inquired. "Is that an addiction?" It could be. We discussed that all binge eaters binge and all food addicts binge, but not all binge eaters are food addicts. The idea is a bit messy to sort, but true. And sort it, Paulina did.

Paulina had to learn how to deal with her eating disorder—particularly her food addiction—and she was able to. The only resolution for Paulina was to stay away from the sugar, flour, and wheat, and then the crazy thinking stopped, and *normalization* ensued.

Have you ever gone back for an extra serving of food when you weren't hungry? What about that last bite when you're so full your stomach is about to explode? I'm sure most of us at some time or another took an additional serving of food. And I'm most certain you were told about the "starving children" and the "clean plate" club. So, often, we eat beyond full. But does this mean you have binge eating disorder? What about food addiction? How do you know?

If you look around, I'm certain you will see at every turn someone who binge eats. Do you? Millions of Americans are stealing, hiding, and hoarding food to secretly binge eat, and after their indulgence are filled with remorse and shame.

One of the least discussed and most common of eating disorders is binge eating disorder. Binge eating is defined as overeating a large amount of food in a short period of time at least three times a week for six months or longer. Binge eating, or compulsive eating, as it is more familiarly known, affects more than twenty million people in the United States alone. And yet we focus more on bulimia and anorexia when considering eating disorders.

In my practice, more than seventy percent of my eating disordered patients suffer from binge eating disorder and/or obesity. This is not to say all bingers are obese or even overweight because some actually can be of normal weight. My biggest challenge is sorting out if the patient has an issue with compulsive eating, or if they have a food addiction, or a combination of both.

Food addiction also has to do with eating a large amount of food in a short period of time, and like compulsive eating, comes with consequences that can be lethal, such as obesity, heart disease, relationship issues, body image, etc.

The big difference between the two disorders is that food addicts crave specific foods and have uncontrollable urges, no matter what they try to do to stop. I liken food addiction and an unmanageable craving for high sugar and processed foods to an addiction to recreational drugs such as cocaine, heroin, and nicotine.

In all cases, the substance-dependent individual consumes larger amounts and for longer periods than was normally intended and has a persistent desire and/or has made repeated unsuccessful attempts to quit...even if the habit interrupts social, recreational, and family interaction as the addicted substance takes precedence in the person's life.

Treatment for binge eating disorder often centers not on the food ***but rather on emotional deficits***. When treatment for food addiction is the issue, on the other hand, ***the***

approach is about the food—and we look at specific foods that trigger the compulsion to consume large amounts of them, no matter what the cost. Binge eating disorder and food addiction show up with many of the same symptoms, though, as food addiction shares the emotional component of binge eating disorder as well as symptoms such as obsession with body, weight, mood shifts, closet eating, and stealing—whereas compulsive eating is about the inability to deal with emotions.

Is Something Wrong with Me?

Above all else, guard your heart, for everything you do flows from it. I suffered from food addiction as far back as I can remember. I just didn't know what it was called. I thought something was wrong with me mentally. I craved chocolate, donuts, chips, and anything gooey and sweet beyond normalcy, and I tried every diet under the sun—including diet pills, commercial diet centers, starvation, over-exercising, and of course indulging in cheat days—none of which helped me tame the compulsion to eat beyond full in spite of the detrimental consequences, which in my case was obesity.

I was broken. Guarding my heart was foreign to me—and for sure everything I did flowed from my heart. In my dysfunction, only negativity was flowing. I was lost, scared, and overwhelmed. Wherever I traveled, I took my food issues with me. No mountain was high enough, no valley low enough, to bring me to my solution with my closed heart and mind. I thought the answer lay in dieting. It did not. The solution starts with confronting the food issue from the core of its foundation.

I wish I knew then what I know now about eating disorders, treatment, and spiritual recovery. Perhaps I could have avoided all the pain and suffering with my weight up and my weight down—an endless battle until now. Today, I live life without the torture of worrying about getting heavy. I no longer crave foods I can't control the amount of; instead, spiritually, my cup is full.

So, if you're one to eat an extra serving, or two, or three, beyond holidays, birthdays, and long weekend temptations, and when you weren't hungry, to the point of devastating consequences that hamper the quality of your life—perhaps you may suffer from an eating disorder.

Do you fit in any of these categories?

My twenty-three years' experience as a clinician, and as one who personally experienced an eating disorder along with food addiction, has not only made me a recognized expert in my field, but also made me privy to understanding the journey of those releasing their obsessions with food and healing from the inside out.

Now that we've examined sugar, salt, and fat in Chapter 11, and food addiction in Chapter 12, exploring how food and mood (Chapter 13) fit into the equation with the cheat days mentality makes sense.

Personal Inventory Questions

1. The food fester is not always a food addict but can be just a foody who gets caught up in eating for entertainment rather than out of hunger or needing nutritional supplies to sustain life. Eating is *a thing to do*. While for most people celebrating with rich foods isn't all about the food, for the food addict it is. Are you a food addict? Is food on your mind 24/7?
2. Proverbs 423: *Above all else, guard your heart, for everything you do flows from it.* Do you guard your heart? How does your heart impact your eating?
3. My getaway is a place where I experienced many, many moments of eating frenzy in my youth. As I've noted elsewhere, Easter particularly was a time to eat and get

carried away with the Cadbury Creme Egg filled with a luscious soft center. Do you have a place that triggers your eating? How can you make your getaway there a positive experience without food taking precedence?

4. So, how do you stop the binge cycle? The first step is to remove the foods that cause you to eat out of control in the first place. Most often those foods are sugar, flour, and wheat. Make a list of the foods that you struggle with for awareness of what the culprits are.
5. Did you know cigarettes contain sugar? And what about potato chips? When you are vigilant, paying attention to the ingredients in your foods, you're on your way to breaking the addiction to food. Take a moment to scout out foods in your pantry, fridge, and freezer that are laced with sugar, flour, and wheat—to confront what's standing between you and your success in beating food addiction.
6. When I first began recovery, I was only dealing with the television commercials to entice me. Now, we have the internet, social media, and other forums screaming EAT ME with their sugar, flour, and wheat-laced foods. What advertisements pull you in? And how can you change that?
7. I love the line in Dr. Livingston's article where he says, "I'll spare you the full story, but let's just say there's probably nothing you've done with food I haven't done myself." What about you? Is this statement true for you? What comes to mind as you read that?
8. Are you a night eater? What thoughts arise for you as you read Betty's story? What steps from the reading speak to you in order to cease this behavior?
9. No surgery is going to remove food addiction. When you read of Paulina's hardships, what part of her story mimics your story?
10. Treatment for binge eating disorder is often not about the food, ***but rather about the emotional deficits.***

Treatment for food addiction ***is about the food***—specific foods trigger the compulsion to consume large amounts of them for that person, no matter what the cost. What are your emotional deficits? What food triggers the compulsion to consume large amounts no matter the cost.

Chapter 13

Food and Mood

Today is the day to break free from
the person you know yourself to be
and step into a self you have yet to know.
Will it be comfortable?
No, but do it anyway.
~Debbie Ford

Certain things we eat cause a shift in mood, especially for those who are sensitive to specific items. The belief that these foods bring happiness is a misreading, as they often cause agitation, cravings, and depression, and possibly set off binge eating.

What are these foods, you might ask. That depends. Food sensitivities are personal, meaning what might bother one person may not trigger another, but for food-addicted individuals, generally sugar, flour, and wheat are the culprits, as described in Chapter 12 on food addiction.

So why bring up food addiction again if we've discussed it? Well, because understanding food addiction and implementing a plan for festive occasions are two different mental processes.

It's one thing to grasp that eating this chocolate tart will create an agitation in your mood, making you irritable or angry, another to counter *gosh this would taste so good, and heck everybody else is eating it.*

The emotional belief is if I don't eat these foods when I'm in Hawaii, or Italy, or Uganda, I won't *feel* the experience of their culture. Or I will miss out. Or worse, I won't have a good time on my trip.

But eating the specific food you're sensitive to, leaving you bloated, and soon your clothes will no longer fit, is a worse experience than missing out on the chocolate tart that everybody else is devouring. *Sometimes we have to feel uncomfortable before we can feel comfortable.* In other words, letting go of the self you were to become the self you want to be isn't always going to feel so good, but as Debbie Ford says, *"Just do it anyway."*

A Jaunt to Vegas

When I was in my early twenties attending DePaul University in Chicago, I worked at an Italian restaurant on the South Side, called, Senese's Winery, an Italian family-owned restaurant. Most of us working there were attending college, working to make ends meet. We became tightly bonded. As such, we decided as a group to go to Las Vegas, where the city never sleeps. I was in awe. Here I was, a wide-eyed kid who'd never ever been to such a place as Vegas.

Prior to the trip, I dieted my way to a few sizes smaller to feel more comfortable in my clothes, and confident, as I was quite shy and insecure. I was visiting Vegas, in all its glitter and charm, embellished wall to wall with talking/beeping slot machines, boasting the biggest names in music, comedy, and more, and with *food—lots and lots of food.*

One hotel after the other was filled with glitz and glamour, and an energy almost indescribable. Who could forget Caesars Palace through the eyes of a twenty-something. This luxury hotel and casino in Paradise, Nevada is situated on the west side of the Las Vegas Strip, between Bellagio (which wasn't there at the time), and The Mirage. It's one of the largest and best-known landmarks in this entertainment and gambling town.

Walking through the casino, goggling at high rollers playing table games such as blackjack, craps, roulette, and poker was truly mind boggling, not to mention watching the slot machines, which strongly attracted me.

I already was knee deep in my undiagnosed eating disorder of binge eating and bulimia through exercise, long before I understood I had food addiction—which was causing my inability to control myself over certain foods. So each time the trays of hors d'oeuvres and drinks came around, I partook.

A few days into our trip, my clothes began to cut into my waistline, leaving a burn mark to the point I couldn't endure the discomfort. I took a portion of my $300 winnings and purchased new blue jeans and other clothes to breathe right again. *I needed to go up two sizes.*

No doubt, food and mood were taking a toll on me as I strolled up and down the strip. The likes of Frank Sinatra, Sammy Davis Jr., Dean Martin, Rod Stewart, Stevie Nicks, to name a few, roamed these very same streets, and perhaps stayed in this very hotel—for sure entertained in it. I was star-struck, feeling myself to be small, insignificant, and inadequate, turning to food to calm my nerves, yet feed my anxiety, followed by bouts of depression. A great trip and horrible trip all rolled into one.

A Honeymoon Gone Sour

Sherry, a patient I saw a good number of years ago, recounted her honeymoon in St. Thomas, sitting out on the balcony, overlooking the restaurant and outdoor bar with the ocean as a backdrop, stuffing her face with chocolate coconut candies she'd picked up at one of the tourist stores.

While looking down at the crowd of people dining, drinking, and dancing, island music flowing upward, she eyed her new husband guzzling shots of whiskey. "How ironic. I'm newly married to the love of my life, and on the first night of our honeymoon, he's getting drunk down below at the outdoor bar, and I'm sitting on the balcony stuffing my mouth with sweet sensations as fast as I can get them in. I could feel my energy lifting from the candies, a euphoric high, yet simultaneously, panic took over at the sight of my husband, slamming down one shot after the other."

Sherry went on to disclose her thought at the time. "We're both sick—really, really sick, and if we don't rein this in, we're doomed before we even start."

Sherry realized she needed help with her food addiction that very night out on the balcony, and in time—with her gentle prompting—her husband, Charlie, identified his alcoholism. Sherry recognized the euphoric feeling she got from eating the sugary concoction but also noted that the high was followed by a low. The rest of their honeymoon circled around drinks and food, with very little lovemaking, or connecting as two newlyweds.

Both Sherry and her husband, Charlie, found their way to therapy, and simultaneously to Food Addicts Anonymous, for Sherry, and Alcoholics Anonymous, for Charlie. Two children, and ten years later, both clean of their addictions, they returned to St. Thomas for a repeat honeymoon, but this time they really took it in.

Sherry and Charlie didn't need the high-calorie, empty-fuel foods or cocktails to indulge in when the island offered so much more. They were now armed and ready to pamper their senses, sans toxic foods and spirits, to experience the ultimate Caribbean. They golfed, hiked, took a thrilling 700-foot skylift to the top of Charlotte Amalie, and rode horses along the shoreline—connecting to each other and their surroundings, unlike the first time they had traveled to this tropical paradise.

No doubt Sherry and Charlie learned that plunging into their addictions affected their moods. This time, they easily found delicious meals that fit their style of healthy eating. They spoiled themselves with lobster, asparagus, and roasted sweet potatoes. They availed themselves of countless options, from breakfast to lunch, and dinner to snacks. They wanted for nothing, except both wishing they'd previously been armed with the awareness they now had on the connection between food and mood, and in Charlie's case, alcohol and mood.

The pictures of their honeymoon, and their revisited, second honeymoon, were very telling regarding the impact the foods and booze had made on this loving couple. In the recent photos, they looked happy and in love, and totally present in picture after picture, whereas on their actual honeymoon they had seemed somber and sad, and were looking off into the distance in photo after photo. Sometimes a picture *is worth a thousand words.*

Food and Mood

Harvard Health Publishing in an article entitled "Food and mood: Is there a connection?" acknowledged that at times digging into a container of ice cream while blindly watching television after a tough day at work might bring comfort—that food and mood are sometimes linked.

The article concurs that stress eating is a verified phenomenon, but states that the actual relationship between food and mood disorders, such as depression, is less clear. Though a concrete answer is less clear, more and more evidence has emerged that a relationship between food and mood does exist.

If we were to ask a food-addicted person, they would agree hands down a correlation is present. And ask any health expert if eating a diet of processed foods is going to give someone an overall stable mood, and again, hands down, the answer will be no. Charlie and Sherry would attest to that without blinking an eye. They knew all too well the living hell processed foods and drink caused in their early years of marriage.

A Trip to the Mediterranean

The Mediterranean diet presents, overall, a healthy, high-quality dietary pattern, not only for promoting a more stable mood but also providing an overall reduction in chronic health conditions. This was the style of eating that fit Charlie and Sherry's life, and most likely yours too.

The Mediterranean diet consists of eating a wide variety of fruits and vegetables, which contain antioxidants that can help reduce inflammation. Imagine a diet of foods like sweet cherries, juicy strawberries, broccoli and leafy green vegetables, and much more of the kind, all foods encouraged on the Mediterranean diet.

Whole grains such as brown rice and quinoa, and rolled oats can be found most places traveled. Olive oil is a huge staple on a clean food plan, along with fish, such as salmon (preferably wild caught), trout, and cod. The list goes on and on, with healthy, delicious *real* foods to be eaten from all parts of the world.

This is not to promote any diets out there called the Mediterranean diet, though they're a fine place to start, but rather the "real" Mediterranean way of eating based on how people eat in that part of the world.

The traditional diet in the countries surrounding the Mediterranean Sea, including France, Italy, Spain, Morocco, and Greece, was once considered a "poor man's" diet, developed over the centuries as people clamored to create sustenance in less hospitable terrain. Today, it is recognized as one of the healthiest ways to eat.

This style of eating offers a great way to replace the saturated fats in the average American diet. The emphasis on fruits, vegetables, lean meats, fish, and other natural foods make up this way of eating. And the bonus is that this way of eating can correct the volatile mood swings of highs and lows created by a diet containing many processed foods.

Have you ever noticed when you've not eaten in a while, you're hungry and angry at the same time (hangry)? Or, have you ever noticed when you eat specific foods, regardless of whether you're hungry or not, they make you either irritable or euphoric? Why is this?

One time, at an eating disorder conference, I heard the speaker say, "Maybe it's no coincidence that food and mood are just a letter apart. The two are peas in a pod." How cleverly put. They do go side by side for those of us who have awakened to the connection.

The speaker went on to say, "Have you ever noticed, on a good day, you eat a large salad with tons of colorful veggies and chunks of chicken, and on a really bad day you eat a tumbler of chocolate-chunk ice cream with dollops of peanut butter, standing at the counter, spoon after spoon after spoon."

Oh my, yes on that one…yes…yes…yes. Or, have you ever had one of those days when you were stuck in traffic and found as soon as your car was moving again, you went to the nearest fast food drive-through for greasy French fried potatoes, and greasy fried chicken nuggets, and maybe even a chocolate shake to top it off? Why? It's because you were looking for comfort food.

A Taste for Comfort

So while Harvard isn't certain enough to commit to whether a connection can be found between food and mood, evident to most of us is that our moods do dictate whether we will indulge in certain foods, and how specific foods make us feel once we ingest them. Now here are two peas in a pod, too—good mood good food, bad mood bad foods…

So imagine yourself on vacation, and everyone seems to be eating decadent foods. Perhaps you're feeling left out, mouthwatering for whatever food experience you believe they're having. Even if you maintain a healthy diet, desiring the high-calorie, unhealthy treats when feeling agitated, stressed, depressed, or left out is normal.

The problem is that *after* the indulgence, reality takes hold. Maybe you were fueling up for fight-or-flight mode because times were getting tough sitting there eating your Mediterranean style of foods while others were chomping on some fried concoction—food otherwise known as comfort foods.

Why do you think they're called *comfort foods*? Because they may make you feel warm and fuzzy at first. They certainly will change your mood for the moment since you're getting what you think you want—*because everybody else is eating it.* But after the treat, you will most likely feel depressed or anxious. Research shows that foods full of fat *and* sugar only increase the likelihood of depression and anxiety, which will lead you to simply want more sugary junk to fight the new bad mood, according to Minati Singh, PhD, of the University of Iowa, in "Food, Mood, and Obesity," a *Frontiers in Psychology* article.

It's a vicious cycle.

According to Singh, food is a potent natural reward, and food intake is a complex process. Reward and gratification are associated with food consumption, which leads to dopamine production, which in turn activates reward and pleasure centers in the brain. She goes on to say an individual will repeatedly eat a particular food to experience this positive feeling of gratification.

However, once we continue this type of repetitive behavior of food intake, the pattern leads to the activation of brain reward pathways that eventually override other signals of satiety and hunger.

In other words, if devouring fats and sugar goes on too long, our body will adapt to it, and think it's normal. Perhaps this is the problem for the majority of people eating processed foods. Maybe this unfortunate way of eating has become "normal." And of course when we try to start eating more nutritiously, we can upset the apple cart, so to speak, causing us to slip into a funk of anxiety or depression and causing an uncontrollable desire for more of the processed foods to feel better—since that's how we've conditioned our bodies. So now we're trapped in a cycle of bad eating in order to try and boost our mood. And we know all too well this is a terrible place to be.

How do you shake this vicious cycle? I'd say begin the process long before you go on your vacation, or weekend getaway, or celebrate your birthday. You can avoid this downward spiral by beginning the process of healthy eating and lifestyle long before you get on that plane, or in that car for your outing.

Three weeks of continuous healthy eating of fruits and vegetables, lean proteins, good sources of fat, and fiber-rich carbohydrates, along with dairy (if you can tolerate it) is a first step in correcting the eating pattern. And soon you'll find a huge dropping away from poor quality eating and shifting to healthy eating. A positive attitude will then surface, and cravings will diminish, if not altogether disappear. Happy days will become your norm…

Many experts (me included) believe that when you're happier from eating healthy foods, you'll want to keep eating healthy foods to recreate the pattern, just as you ate poor quality foods because that was your habit. We can rewrite the script by eating healthier no matter where we are, who we're with, or what's going on in our lives. We don't need to have a food fest frenzy to have fun, or fit in, or belong. I promise.

I would be remiss to not mention hypoglycemia here—low blood sugar, which for sure affects food and mood, and can be tricky when trying to travel.

Managing Hypoglycemia, Food Addiction, and Travel

I'm on a Zen-like getaway in the township of Mt. Morris, which hovers next to Wautoma, Wisconsin, taking in the quiet sounds of nature while sitting on the porch at the cabin, writing this piece on food and mood and about my airport experience with food, in total serenity. The smell of pine trees, tree frogs calling out to each other, birds singing, along with a cool summer breeze, blend into a perfect recipe for Zen. Life is good.

And then, crunch…crunch, CRUNCH…I'm not alone! I look up abruptly, expecting a big black grizzly bear, as I know they're out here. But the animal I spot is a deer, sporting an impressive rack of antlers. Our eyes lock. Neither of us moves. Looking deep into his golden brown eyes, I connect for what seems like forever. We're so close, I can almost feel his breath.

Darn, no phone to capture our moment. Slowly, I rise to snatch my phone from indoors, and in a blink of an eye he's gone. Graceful, picking each step, he slips into the forest.

Okay…back to my story. Recently at the Fort Lauderdale Airport, I was trying to look inconspicuous, balancing my large food bag, carry-on luggage, and a ginormous gold bag, hoping to pass it off as my purse. Before I got too far, an elderly TSA agent, coal black eyes peering up over his glasses, arm extended, blocking me sternly—the only thing missing being a whistle—said, "Ma'am, you have three bags, only two allowed."

I gulped, flushed red, as my food bag tumbled off my shoulder, and I wobbled to balance my oversized purse and luggage. Quickly regrouping, without hesitation, I told him the third bag was food, that I have hypoglycemia. Instantly, he softened, morphing into a grandfatherly fella waving me through.

I'm a food addict in recovery and suffer with hypoglycemia, so packing food essentials is critical. But, the amazing "cheap" tickets required only one personal and one carry-on. ***Not three bags***—the third would house my food. I took it anyway. Fear engulfed me, thinking they'd make me put one to the side or check it in, neither of which I wanted to do.

Okay, so you say, *what's the big deal of checking my bag?* Big deal is I'm on a split travel, and need to grab my bags quickly to make my connection in twenty minutes. Yes, tight for sure. I feared one of the bags would be left behind. I purchased the most amazing tickets, but they came with this challenge. A large, checked-in suitcase can house all my essentials, including food. Not so with a carry-on bag—the maximum dimensions are nine by fourteen by twenty-two inches, including handles and wheels.

So what was the issue? I had to carry my foods and clothes for my reunion with classmates I hadn't seen in a hundred years—or at least it felt that way.

Anyway, I have hypoglycemia, also known as low blood sugar—where blood sugar decreases to below normal levels, which can lead to a wide variety of symptoms including clumsiness, trouble talking, confusion, loss of consciousness, seizures, and even death. A feeling of hunger, sweating, shakiness, and weakness may also be present.

To avoid all that discomfort, I travel with foods in my luggage *and* in my lunch bag, but this time, I was loaded down with clothes and toiletries for six days, including an outfit for my class reunion, leaving no space.

Bringing all my foods was essential. When my blood symptoms come on quickly, they don't recede. The feeling is awful, and I ward it off by eating at regular intervals, avoiding hunger or long periods without food.

Hypoglycemia can be caused by medications to treat diabetes mellitus, kidney failure, certain disorders such as insulinoma, liver disease, hypothyroidism, starvation, inborn error of metabolism, severe infections, reactive hypoglycemia, as well as the effect of a number of drugs, including alcohol.

Low blood sugar can occur in otherwise healthy persons who haven't eaten in several hours. A quick treatment is to eat foods high in simple sugars. With low blood sugar, clean foods at hand to avoid the dip are crucial. One time, I was told I couldn't bring my food bag, as I had too many bags. I left my food behind, but a few hours into my flight I felt nauseas, confused, irritable, and lethargic, needing attendance. Lesson learned. Now I know I need to say my food is for medicinal purposes. And I'm good to go.

So, there I was at the airport, waiting to pass through the TSA. I had so much stuff, luggage items were spilling out of my "personal" bag. The outcome might have been a repeat if I had been told no. Speaking up is important— those with hypoglycemia need to be vigilant and proactive.

So, you're saying as you read this, hey just pack less and you'll avoid the problem. I agree. Lesson learned this time—I hope.

I determined long ago that my priority must be my food; money, ID, phone, and laptop—everything else—can be ditched.

Remedies for Low Blood Sugar: Real Food

Symptoms include:

- Tiredness
- Increased appetite
- Cloudy thinking
- Blurry vision
- Inability to concentrate
- Pale complexion
- Sweating

The hypoglycemic state is almost an "out of body "experience. I begin to slip away, becoming really quiet…and quite moody. The most common treatment is glucose tablets, but food addicts can't eat sugar glucose tablets, which are chalky, white, dry tablets that work within minutes to restore blood sugar levels. As a food addict, I don't consider sugar an option. I prefer natural treatment—*real food.*

Real Food Treatment

1. **Food.** Never leave it to chance. Vigilance, preparing your food in advance to avoid being left without your foods, is a first step.
2. **Eat at Regular Intervals.** Not only carrying your food is essential to stopping the symptoms of low blood sugar, but also eating at regular intervals is key. Eating every four to five hours works for me, but for you the timing might be every three hours.

3. **All-natural Peanut Butter.** Real peanut butter with no added sugar is easy to tote and eat, and provides quick relief. Stores such as Whole Foods, or those offering organic foods, often carry small, pre-measured packets of peanut butter, making it easier to transport during your travels or outings.
4. **Dry Fruits.** Raisins, pineapple, mango, and dates are a few very sweet fruits that will instantly pull you out of the funk before it gets out of hand. Make sure to check ingredients as some companies pack these with sugar. The only ingredient on the label should be the fruit itself.
5. **Applesauce.** Fresh applesauce, either homemade or store bought, is another easy, doable food. Again, some companies package individual-sized applesauce portions, making it easier to take with you. Or homemade is always a guarantee; it's, for sure, natural without sugar.
6. **Fresh Fruits.** Banana is the first that comes to mind. You can find a banana at just about any store, gas station, or fresh food market. They're affordable and easy to put in your purse/bag. Grapes and pineapple are sweet fruits that can also put a quick stop to the symptoms once they start.
7. **Grapes.** Red or green grapes are a simple fix and easy to carry. Pop a few in your mouth and you're good to go.
8. **Pineapple.** Fresh pineapple is one of the sweetest fruits sure to help you bounce back.
9. **Dried fruits.** As a backup to store in your purse or bag, turn to dry fruits as a constant. Instead of white, chalky sugar tablets, go natural. Dried fruits will keep for many weeks and are great to have on hand.
10. **Eat at Regular Intervals.** This advice is worth repeating—you can avoid the slump and needing any of the above real food fixes if you eat at regular four to five hour intervals.

Get to know your body and your symptoms to offset them before they hit. Eating every four hours—at most five—slows or stops the problem from coming on.

Food addiction is real—and recovery is possible if you're vigilant. And hypoglycemia or low blood sugar is real, too, but can be offset when you're prepared. I'm vigilant…and have been eating clean for the past twenty-plus years, but at times in my earlier years of recovery, I took a chance and left my "treatments" behind, thinking all would be well. Sometimes, though, you might be caught in an unforeseeable situation—like stuck in traffic for hours, on a plane or train—or trapped in any other situation.

Stay true to yourself, practice self-love and self-care, and you'll sail through your low blood sugar and food addiction without a miss.

Dr. Lisa's Personal Quick Fix, Self-love, and Self-care Formula:

1. Let go of sugar, flour, and wheat.
2. Exercise daily, or close to it.
3. Drink water.
4. Meditate.
5. Pray.
6. Laugh and smile.
7. Connect with others.
8. Breathe
9. Eat real food; never leave it to chance.
10. Take supplements

In the stillness, I'm writing away. The only sounds are of birds chatting back and forth in different octaves, and the chirping of crickets—all else are asleep after a long day. My class reunion was one of the highlights of my trip—seeing friends, sharing memories and life's journeys over the past forty-five years. Wrapping up my thoughts, I feel eyes on me. This time I only raise my eyes. My buck friend and I stare, once again communicating without words.

What about your birthday? Tune in to Chapter 14 for ways to maneuver around your special day without sinking into the sugar abyss.

Personal Inventory Questions

1. Do you recognize that certain foods cause you a euphoric mood, while others make you feel sad and upset? Is it possible you have a food/mood connection? Explore what identifying which foods bring you difficulty might look like for you.
2. Today is the day to break free from the person you know yourself to be and step into a self you have yet to know (Debbie Ford). Who do you know yourself to be? And what self will you step into that you have yet to know? Would you like to be a person comfortable with your food plan wherever you go—even if at first the transition is uncomfortable?
3. The emotional belief is if I don't eat these foods when I'm in Hawaii, or Italy, or Uganda, I won't *feel* the experience of their culture. Or I'll miss out. Or worse, I won't have a good time on my trip. Are these your thoughts? Many share this same emotional belief system. What would it be like for you to be anywhere in the world under any circumstances and to eat the foods that are your foods, and pass on the ones that aren't?
4. Have you ever dieted to a lower weight, knowing you were going on a trip the way I did prior to my trip to Vegas? Why do you think we do that? What was your experience like? Did you have to buy larger clothes for your return?

5. What do you think about Sherry on her honeymoon, hiding out in their room and eating as fast as she could shovel in food, while her husband, Charlie, was down below in the outside bar near the ocean drinking himself into oblivion? Have you ever done such a thing as Sherry—or Charlie?
6. Harvard Health Publishing, in an article entitled "Food and mood: Is there a connection?" acknowledges at times digging into a container of ice cream while blindly watching television after a tough day at work might bring comfort—that food and mood are sometimes linked. Do you find after a troubling day, you indulge to counteract your rough day—or on a long weekend, or vacation for that matter?
7. The Mediterranean diet promotes healthy veggies, lean protein, good sources of fat, and high fiber carbs, along with dairy, as food staples best to promote optimal health. What are your thoughts? How close to this style of eating do you find yourself?
8. Often others around you will be eating high-calorie foods that you might be quite sensitive to. Or perhaps you know these foods to be "comfort" foods. Might you add new healthy foods to your list that could promote comfort and overall health as well?
9. Do you suffer from low blood sugar—hypoglycemia? What are some takeaways from this section that you can work into your healthy lifestyle?
10. Food, the right food, is key to making travel successful. How are you practicing your self-love and self-care when you don't feel good?

Part III

Turn the Corner

Chapter 14

It's My Birthday!!

The moment I have realized God
sitting in the temple of every human body,
The moment I stand in reverence
before every human being
and see God in him—
That moment I am free from bondage,
everything that binds vanishes, and I am free.
~Swami Vivekananda~

Within each of us rests our Higher Source—our creator—in you, in me, and in others—and *the moment I stand in reverence before every human being and see God in him—that moment I am free from bondage, everything that binds vanishes, and I am free.*

Your birthday, a day commemorating the birth of you, marks the beginning of your life on earth. Most cultures celebrate a person on their date of birth. The birth of you is a day about you, a day to honor your very arising to participate in life.

The anniversary of the birth of you is a day for you to be thankful for what you've done thus far with your life—perhaps your accomplishments, or any talents that you may have been gifted with. But the anniversary of a birth day is more than your accumulations, it's day to appreciate your opportunity to live. As time marches on, though, birthdays have an increasingly bad rap in terms of…ageing…getting old…fear of illness…a time some don't want to acknowledge at all—they're not proud to add another year. We forget, or don't realize, God is sitting in the temple of everybody, including our own.

Or maybe all your loved ones have passed and you're alone, or your children are estranged from you, or you have bad memories. This, no doubt, is tough.

I recall when I was a child and I was about to turn twelve years old, my mother became very involved in marching and giving to the poor. She was palling around with the likes of Father Leonard Feeney, a well-known priest, later defrocked by the Vatican in 2005 for alleged sexual misconduct.

Fr. Feeney was the brother of the Joe Feeney I mentioned earlier who took the accordion gig on Lawrence Welk, the very one my dad turned down—they never met. Coincidentally, my mom befriended the priest brother many years later.

At around this time, at the tail end of my eleventh year, Mom stopped piling gifts under the Christmas tree, and birthdays went unnoticed. A wonderful spiritual gesture, indeed, but not so easy to understand when you're a kid with no presents, no cake, and no party. I was confused and hurt—but never voiced my feelings, fearing I was bad for having such thoughts.

The first year as an adult that I didn't partake in cake, many thought this wasn't "natural," that this was my birthday, and cake was okay…just this once. Others seemed more disturbed than I over the issue of not eating cake. But this time the decision not to eat cake was mine, unlike when I was a child and birthdays disappeared.

Every completed birth year gives us an occasion to rethink how we're living our lives thus far. That anniversary of our birth doesn't have to be a food-fest celebrated with rich cakes and thick icing.

No Cake!

I recall a mom sitting on the couch in front of me at my office during a session with her daughter, who suffered from binge eating disorder and food addiction, tears streaming down her face, as her daughter announced that she didn't want a cake for her birthday. Mom was quite upset. How can you have a birthday without cake? The idea is deeply engraved in us that cake and gifts must accompany the celebration of a person's birth. Is that so? Really?

What about regarding your birth date, your birth day, as a refresher, a do-over prospect, or a chance to regenerate, mentally, physically, and spiritually.

Perhaps your birthday can provide a time to reflect on what this life has brought you—the gift of life itself.

Every year on my birthday now, I journal my goals for the year—a rebirth, or reset if you will. I see this time as a break to map out how to live each blessed day, 86,400 seconds to be exact, that's been given.

Okay, so you're thinking yeah, yeah, that's good, but what about the party, the gifts, the balloons, the family gathering, and all that. Well, those can be positives too. Celebrating with friends and family is wonderful, but what about giving a gift to someone else on your birthday…and often the most precious gifts received are the ones made from the heart.

That honoring of our birth doesn't have to be about what's spent, or what's eaten, but can simply provide a moment when we're grateful for another day to experience life. Does the cake really make the event? Or might our natal day be about the people and the connections?

Okay, we're conditioned to believe a birthday isn't "right" if it's not filled with goodies to eat. So what about filling it with healthy goodies?

What would or could a healthy goody be? You could bake a carrot cake made from natural ingredients or muffins made with fruit and oats—or how about yogurt ice cream as mentioned earlier? Get creative, and free yourself from the idea that sugar is going to do the trick. The sugar isn't really what you crave. After so many years of talking to people about these things, I know that what the relentless sugar eaters are after is filling the empty spots in their hearts. Might that apply to you as well?

Melissa lamented, "I can't skip cake for my birthday, it's un-American!" She carried an extra fifty pounds on her petite five-foot-two frame. In addition, she made cakes for a living. She was invested in the idea that celebrations, of any sort, must have cake with thick icing. Melissa claimed she loved food too much to give up any of it, adding that dieting made her utterly miserable.

After a lengthy discussion over several weeks, we unveiled that the way she was approaching this *diet* concept was wrong. Contrary to popular belief, healthy eating doesn't have to be boring. In fact, with a bit of careful management, you can still eat many of your favorite foods. Rather than completely cutting out treats, why not work in some made with real foods. An abundance of healthy foods are out there, so shop around for those that you actually enjoy eating. You may be surprised, the way Melissa was, what you might find.

One recipe loved by all in her family was Melissa's skillet fries:

Ingredients:

- 3 medium potatoes, sliced
- 1 large onion
- 3-4 large vegetables: Bell peppers, sweet peppers, zucchini, eggplant, whole green beans, and carrots all work.
- A pound of beef, chicken, or shrimp chunks, depending on your taste buds.

Instructions:

1. Preheat oven to 425.
2. Rough-chop all the vegetables into 1" cubes.
3. In heated cast iron pan dressed with 2 tablespoons of olive oil, sauté the veggies on medium, until slightly browned.
4. Remove from pan and set aside, return pan to stove and set on high.
5. Add enough olive oil to the pan to cover the bottom.
6. Using a mandolin, slice your potatoes into fries, and quickly add your protein choice to hot oil.
7. Fry potatoes and protein until browned, turning frequently.
8. Drain excess hot oil from pan (caution: it will be VERY hot).
9. When fries are fully browned, add the veggies back to the pan, and pop into oven for about 10 minutes or until fries and protein choices are completely cooked through.
10. Serve and enjoy!

And for Melissa's cake…drum roll…

Melissa discovered this low-carb and sugar-free delight while tooling around the internet searching for a healthy birthday cake option. She found one in which the family wouldn't be able to detect zucchini hidden in the folds of decadent chocolate.

Please keep in mind if you're sensitive to chocolate, this might not be the recipe for you. Some who eliminate sugar, flour, and wheat also eliminate chocolate, a gray-area food.

Know your sensitivities before you indulge. I'm fine with quality dark chocolate, but I abstain from alcohol of any source, another gray-area food. You may be the opposite. The only one who knows you is you! For me, I find alcohol causes cravings and leaves me wanting foods that are processed. My last alcoholic drink was twenty-three years ago; I don't miss it, not one inch.

As for the amount of chocolate, I personally would shave a tiny bit on top of the baked cake to melt, and forgo all frostings. But again, finding your right place is a journey for *you*. Know yourself so you can carve out a "perfect fit" type of eating that is sustainable and doable in your view.

Melissa, grinning from ear to ear, shares that this cake is very simple and quick to prepare. She boasts that it has *real* zucchini, which makes the cake super rich, and moist.

Before starting, you'll need two bowls: one for the dry ingredients (coconut flour, cocoa power, and baking powder) and another for the wet ingredients (eggs, sweetener, vanilla extract) Make sure to mix the wet and the dry ingredients separately and then join them. Once complete, you'll add the shredded zucchini.

Zucchini Chocolate Cake—a two bowl marvel:

Prep time: 10 minutes
Cook Time 30 to 40 minutes
Servings: 12 slices
Ingredients:

- 4 eggs
- ½ stick of butter melted

- 4 tablespoons almond milk
- 1 cup shredded zucchini
- 2/3 cup almond flour
- 1/3 cup coconut flour
- ½ cup cocoa powder
- ½ cup stevia, or any sweetener of your choice
- 1 teaspoon baking powder

Chocolate Frosting (optional)

- 200 grams dark chocolate (no- to low-sugar—under 3grams)
- 3 tablespoons butter
- 4 tablespoons milk

Instructions for Chocolate Zucchini Cake

1. In a large bowl, mix the coconut flour, cocoa powder, stevia, and baking powder.
2. Add the eggs, melted butter, and almond milk. Mix well.
3. Pour the batter into the greased pan and bake at 180°C/360° F for about 30 to 40 minutes, or until a toothpick comes out from the center clean.
4. Allow the cake to cool in the pan for 5 minutes before transferring to a wire rack to cool completely.
5. For the optional frosting, microwave all ingredients for about 2 minutes, stirring a few times throughout cooking time.
6. Once the chocolate zucchini cake is cooled, add the optional frosting and slice into pieces.

Notes

- ✓ If the batter is too thick, add an extra tablespoon or two of liquid.
- ✓ Serves 12

- ✓ 197 calories per serving
- ✓ If wondering, one serving piece equals: 25% fat; cholesterol 33%; total carbohydrates 4%; protein 12%
- ✓ If you count food groups, one serving piece equals: 1 serving of miscellaneous, ¼ protein, 1 fat, ¼ c. milk

If the first frosting option seems too decadent and perhaps too tempting, you might want an Applesauce Chocolate Frosting 4 Ingredient wonder—THE go-to chocolate frosting.

Ingredients:

- Unsweetened applesauce
- Dark cocoa powder
- Coconut oil
- A sticky sweetener of choice—a no-sugar option is monk fruit
- Time needed: 5 minutes

Instructions: Simply sir the ingredients

1. Start by using 1 cup of unsweetened applesauce.
2. Slowly add in the remaining ingredients.
3. Using a teaspoon, add more applesauce slowly, as a little extra can turn the frosting from smooth to soupy.
4. If you want a sweeter chocolate frosting, you can add the monk fruit.

Hint: You can prep this frosting in advance. If you plan on using it on the same day, keep it at room temperature. If you refrigerate it, you'll need to let it thaw out and soften before spreading. You may also need a little extra applesauce to get it moving again. It will count toward your fruit option.

Birthdays don't have to be difficult when you look at them through a different lens. *The moment I have realized God sitting in the temple of every human body, the moment I stand in reverence before every human being and see God in him—that moment I am free from bondage, everything that binds vanishes, and I am free (Swami Vivekananda).*

To date, Melissa has released fifty pounds, maintaining a weight that works for her small frame. She continues to put together decadent meals, but all from the framework of healthy eating, and using real ingredients.

Moving forward, let's travel together through the grocery store as we turn the page to Chapter 15. Come shop with me. Be truly free…

Personal Inventory Questions

1. What do birthdays signify to you? Do you make excuses why you need to eat this or that during this celebratory event?
2. As time marches on, birthdays get a bad rap…ageing…getting old …fear of illnesses…a time some don't want to honor at all. Where do you stand in this? How does it impact you?
3. The birth of you is a day to be thankful for what you've done thus far with your life, perhaps accomplishments or talents that you may have been blessed with. Tally up what's been good so far.
4. We forget, or don't realize, God sitting in the temple of everybody, including our own. Did you forget? How does including your understanding of a Higher Source work in favor for you? Or not?
5. Or maybe all your loved ones have passed, and you're alone, or your children are estranged from you, or you have bad memories. This, no doubt, is tough. Who is missing, and how does this impact you?

6. Do you have great memories or terrible ones relating to your childhood birthdays? Do these memories play a role in how you deal with life's celebrations today?
7. Can you imagine celebrating a birthday without cake?
8. What lovely meal can you create as your "signature meal" for a special day such as a birthday?
9. What thoughts came to mind as your read Melissa's story?
10. Perhaps a meal such as Melissa's can work for you, too. What impact does her idea of celebrating with a special meal have on you?

Chapter 15

Come Shop with Me

One cannot think well, love well, sleep well,
if one has not dined well.
~Virginia Woolf, A Room of One's Own

Food is the key to wellbeing in every respect. So true that one cannot love well, think well, or sleep well, if one has not dined well. Virginia Woolf was spot on. And one of the ways to insure you dine well is to have the right foods with you whether you're home, on vacation, or even in another country.

How can I do this, you might ask. The answer is, through preparation. If you prepare to fail, you will fail, but if you prepare to win, you will win at managing your food, regardless of where you are.

You might be saying, "But I don't have the money to eat well, or to travel, for that matter. So I turn to fast food for the little bit of enjoyment I can find in life." Sounds dismal, but this is something I often hear from patients working through their body, weight, and food challenges. But the situation doesn't have to be that way. Let's look at food and then money to see why I believe so.

First, we'll explore the issue of food and clearing your palate, and then move into money. Who doesn't like to talk about money?

Okay, your palate. How does palate—your preference for certain tastes—factor into food festivities? Clearing your palate might seem like drudgery at first, but once your desire for certain foods is erased, the process of eating well will actually be easy, since you'll soon crave real foods instead of processed foods. Right now, you may be attracted to processed foods because they taste good to you—but I assure you, when your diet is cleared of toxic foods, you'll want to eat foods that are clean and real.

To be clear, when referencing cleansing the palate, I'm not referring to some hoity-toity, fancy way of living that most of us can't relate to, but rather to introducing real foods into your food repertoire—as opposed to the high-fat, sugary, and salty foods I described in Chapter 9.

Anything you put into your mouth can stimulate your taste buds, which are tiny receptors that respond to different types of flavors such as sweet, salty, spicy, pungent, sour, etc. I'm not referring to cleansing the palate from spicy foods or even sweet foods or removing the taste of coffee by covering it over with a subtle taste of cream. What I'm talking about is when you're feeding predominantly on rich, processed foods, you acquire a taste for those foods.

At first, any foods that are natural may seem bland and undesirable to eat. Once you're clear, however, you'll actually taste the succulent richness in real food, and this won't take a long time to accomplish, either. A sweet pepper will taste sweet, whereas once it didn't. An orange will now yield its sweet-sour citric taste with a dash of sour in its juicy and chewy texture. That orange, you'll discover, offers a burst of flavors, waking up your taste buds, something you might not have noticed before.

Salads of romaine and iceberg lettuces will crunch, and adding watercress and arugula will contribute a peppery bite, with more to be desired—where before, maybe not so much as compared to fried foods with salt and fat as the tease. But now, slowing down the eating and savoring each bite of *real food* will open up tastes you didn't pay attention to before.

So to cleanse your palate is to let go of those "manufactured" foods and replace them with real, non-processed foods. Once you're clear, you'll taste foods in a whole different way, enjoying bursts of flavor you never knew existed. The taste when you compare the processed to unprocessed foods is amazing.

Small Packages Are the "In" Thing

The other night during dinner, my husband, older son, and I began to discuss foods, packaging, and cost-effective shopping. I went into my rant regarding how food is a necessity for sustaining life, and how for the food-challenged person, food is ominous and frightening, as they have to face dining four times a day, including a half-meal—or snack as some call it.

My son said something like, "The millennials don't like to buy big packages of foods, but rather go for the smaller package." His understanding, from a news report he'd heard earlier that day, was that the younger population isn't prone to stock up on foods. The story said that they prefer teeny packages rather than to buy in bulk. For them, spending money on smaller was okay. I couldn't wrap my brain around this concept. Buying smaller packages isn't cost effective, for sure.

I found this most interesting since I need to have a full fridge, freezer, and pantry to feel safe—as without these I fret that I might go hungry. This stems from my early twenties when I was quite broke and knee deep in my food addiction, and feared to stock an abundance of food, worrying that I'd then binge eat. My best friend, Yvonne, marveled at the fact I only had a jar of peanut butter, a head of lettuce, and skim milk in the fridge. At that time, I thought the less food you had in the home, the less risk of overeating.

Wrong.

A filled pantry, fridge, freezer, and now a deep freezer I've added to the mix, bring great peace and calm to me because I know I have food to eat at all times. A plentiful supply of edibles lessens my fear of not having enough to eat. So I've swung from the fear of having any food at all in the house to oversupplying. Perhaps this need for abundance stems from being the youngest of six children, and Mom tending to others first…maybe. And the skimpy selection definitely arose from the fear of getting fat.

But having said that, for sure the necessity for more food stems from years of chronic dieting. At times I was so hungry I could have chomped on tree bark to fill my stomach. I hopped from one diet to the next, a definite ingredient in binge eating and the dread of not having enough to eat.

So, not only are we working on changing our relationship with food, but we're looking at shopping together now, to make certain you buy enough quality food to eat at a price that makes sense. Yes, that money part again. But hang on…more to say before we look at money abundance, and its connection to food.

So here we were at the dinner table, and I began to ponder *why is it* the younger generation doesn't stock up on food? Is the reason that they're transient—or are they perpetually broke? Or perhaps they eat out at restaurants more often than at home?

I was watching television the other day, a rare treat, and what did I see but a commercial showing peanut butter cups, pointing to how thin they now are—and promoting that this was a desired, good feature for the consumer. As an advocate for saving money and time, I'm thinking, *But then they receive less of it for the same price, so how can that be good.*

This made me think about Kris at the dinner table, saying smaller portions are the "in" thing these days. My mind wandered to the small popcorn and chip bags, and the tiny peanut butter containers promoted at all the supermarkets as well as the club stores such as Sam's Club, BJ's, and Costco, and I thought perhaps this was a ploy to manipulate us consumers into believing less is more.

Or perhaps the strategy is to appeal to us to save calories. You know, the 100-calorie bag of chips, cookies, popcorn, etc. The approach is as if the advertisers are saying we can't be trusted to portion out the exact amount we need from a larger—more cost-effective—package.

But being the money-conscious person I am (*The Millionaire Next Door*!), I think buying in bulk is much more efficient. Why not buy the ginormous bag of Skinny Popcorn and divide it into smaller zip-locked portions yourself? Or what about popping it from its raw version yourself at home and then divide that into portions?

I've given many talks and presentations that revolve around the cost of eating clean and healthy. I often hear from patients and attendees at these talks that only the rich can eat clean and healthy—but I beg to differ. Or I hear eating clean is time consuming or they don't cook. Or how about "After I worked so hard all week, now you want me to cook on the weekends too?" The best excuse I hear is "Why would I go on a vacation and look for a grocery store? *I'm on vacation!!*"

I get it, really I do. But if your goal is to live like no one else so you can live like no one else (words of Dave Ramsey, the Christian finance guru) then shopping for your foods and preparing your foods is one of the first steps. You see, I find those struggling with money are often struggling with their food issues too. Somehow, dollars and calories go hand in hand. In 2011, I noted my food intake relationship began to change when I began the debt free quest. I began to eat less and spend less. I became debt-free on 11-11-11 (yes, I'm a numbers girl).

What's Money (Calories Too) Got to Do with It?

I was sitting pondering a chapter for my upcoming book (this one) on releasing the obsession with cheat days and food fest(s)—fests meaning festivities such as birthdays, weekends, long weekends, holidays, and traveling, events filled with food, and my mind began to drift to thoughts of how much my life changed when I became debt free.

Okay, you say, what the heck does money have to do with breaking free from celebration eating? Well, once upon a time I was broke. Yes, I mean so broke and so in debt I should have been shaking in the knees. For some reason, I wasn't. My inner self told me I'd find my way out.

And I did.

In 1998 I began reading books like *Don't Worry, Make Money: Spiritual and Practical Ways to Create Abundance and More Fun in Life*, and I became a disciple of Dave Ramsey, reading his *Total Money Makeover: A Proven Plan for Financial Fitness* and *The Millionaire Next Door*, along with *Think and Grow Rich*, and many more that would take pages to enumerate. At the same time, I was working my way out of my food addiction—and somehow I began to notice similarities.

In what way? you might ask.

Well, I began to see that I was spending money on total junk food, and that was costing me a fortune. I was eating at every donut shop, stopping at the store to buy poor quality food, and grabbing a coffee laced with cream and sweetener, along with candy bars, at every gas stop—and of course all went on the credit card, with interest in the background eating away at my money every second.

After reading money books, I began to understand that I wasn't respecting my money. I had student debt nearing $300,000, plus a mortgage, car payment, and credit card debt. I was up to my eyeballs in total debt—and I was starting to gain the hundred pounds back I'd lost, because of out-of-control binge eating.

When I took a step back, and began to look at my spending and my eating, I had a revelation…an aha moment—and realized the two went hand in hand, and if I worked on the money, I'd probably get a grip on the food.

I did!

I began to write down every morsel of food I was eating, and every dollar I was spending—at the same time working on Dave Ramsey's Snowball idea…paying down my smallest credit card, and working my way up. Eventually, I saw light at the end of the tunnel. Every time I paid off a credit card, I had that much more money to throw at the next card…on and on…until I paid off all my cards, and then moved on to the car…then the STUDENT LOAN, which was enough to choke a horse.

After nibbling away at the other debts, the money I then had to throw at this debt became enormous. *I lived poor so that I could live rich.*

When I freed myself from the student loan, I went all out and paid off the house mortgage, and to date I live debt free. **Debt Free!!** And my food bill is not enormous because I learned to buy real foods in bulk…and store them in the freezer, and pantry, and divvy them out in pre-made packages.

You can do this too.

If you're drowning in debt, and your weight is climbing, you, too, can take a step back, work toward eating clean and healthy and letting go of your debts, and watch the magic happen. Buy books on managing money or check them out of the library, and learn to eat real foods, and life will become a whole lot better.

And the funny thing is that when you practice working toward becoming debt free, and then living debt free, you actually thereafter stay in a frugal way of living. But…when you want to go on that vacation, or you want to buy that piece of jewelry, or you're ready for a new car, you buy it in cash, and don't feel the dent.

A favorite quote of mine from Richard Carlson's ***Don't Worry, Make Money: Spiritual and Practical Ways to Create Abundance and More Fun in Your Life*** is "One of the most severely limiting beliefs that many of us have is that the person we were yesterday is the person we have to be today." Not so. If you hang onto this type of belief system, you will remain heavy, addicted to foods—and perhaps broke. The idea that you can't be a different person is a self-defeating belief, which goes against the self-love and self-care I speak of in this very book you're reading.

What do you think? Do you see a correlation between your consumed calories and your financial status? Examine this interrelationship closely, and see if you can find ways to change your belief system. Having more money isn't about how much money you make, but rather about how much you save. And losing weight isn't about how many calories you eat, but rather how much *quality* food you consume.

Perhaps you started this book diet driven, financially shaky, overweight, and in desperate need of a makeover. Perhaps you want to travel, but you fear clothes won't fit, money is lacking, and you need to start your diet first. Stop that thinking now. You're beautiful as you are.

Save Big—Shop in Bulk

Shop in bulk at a "club" type store to save a good thirty percent roaming the aisles for only *real* food, steering away from processed and packaged foods. Think natural; think free of sugar, flour, and wheat; think quality fats, protein, veggies, fruit, and dairy, and starchy carbs—and you are more than on your way.

Shopping at a Sam's Club or Costco in bulk—real foods, of course—is much more efficient than going out to a fast food restaurant. I recall in my binge eating days, before I read *The Millionaire Next Door,* stopping at Miami Subs and buying a giant tuna sub, a bag of baked chips, and a Diet Coke. At the time, I thought that was healthy eating. The cost was over ten dollars, and this was years, and years, and years ago.

Had I gone to the store and purchased the tuna and fixings, and a large bag of baked chips, portioned out, along with a tumbler of crushed-ice water with a wedge of lemon, the cost would have been less than a few bucks. We don't have to spend tons of money to eat clean.

I have a generic list of "must haves" that I purchase and stock at all times. First, I always have eggs on hand. Eggs are a versatile protein that can be eaten in a wide variety of ways, such as boiled, poached, and scrambled, which are the basics—but expand your mind. You can make vegetable omelets, muffins, pancakes, etc. with eggs. So yes, eggs are a staple, as are: almond milk, spinach, spring salad mix, bananas, strawberries, apples, oat bran, old fashioned oatmeal, chicken, salmon, cod, lean hamburger, olive oil, avocado oil, and coconut oil, to name a few must-have items.

But what about organic foods you might ask? Well, yes, that's another thing, and I agree organic can be quite costly. I admire those who can afford to purchase from an organic venue, but I choose not to. Yes, if I can buy at a farm market I'm in, but if I'm going to pay triple the amount for the food,

I'm not. I'll buy fresh, and real, but maybe not always organic. A part of me always questions how organic is the organic? Isn't the field still receiving rainwater from the pesticide-laced soil next door? And pollution in the air, isn't it moving from one field to the next? Again, if I can buy organic at a trendy farmers market at reasonable cost, I'm all in.

Our son Benjamin and his wife, Zoe, a lawyer and dietitian respectively, eat very clean, and as organic as they can—but not always. They have their own little garden in the yard, with fresh tomatoes, cucumbers, peppers, rosemary, and other delights. Yay, good for them! I admire these two because they don't fit the millennial way of thinking, as Kris described at the dinner table.

Benjamin and Zoe are savers and economize at all times, yet they travel, go on getaway weekends, cruise, and travel abroad, always on a budget, and eating the best, yet cleanest and most economical foods available. They bought a home and carry out do-it-yourself projects when they can. They caught the wave to *live like no one else, so they can live like no one else.*

A Palate Correction

I recall a time in my life when I ate mostly donuts, cakes, and candy. I also became very sick as I compromised my immune system. I broke out in boils because I was nutritionally deprived. When I thought to eat a piece of fruit, it didn't appeal to me, because my palate was accustomed to salty, rich foods. Real foods tasted bland, and were uninteresting to me.

In time, my palate began to shift, and I could taste the sweetness in a peach and the tart in the lemon. Food—real food—burst with flavor in my mouth for the first time. I began to crave fruits and vegetables, leaving no desire for processed foods. The shift was huge for me, and will be huge for you.

At one time grocery shopping was frightening for me, as my cart automatically traveled down the middle aisles where the cookies, cakes, and candies lurk. One time I automatically went down my customary aisles, shaking with fear as I powered my way down each row, attempting not to toss my old staples of junk foods in my cart. The trip down the aisle was hard.

In time, I learned not to go down those aisles and worked off of a list of foods that were my new go-tos. Many times I also had to put back foods that were "impulse" grabs, as I was transitioning to this new way of eating. But transition I did.

I now make my way down the outer aisles of the store. I don't need anything elsewhere for the most part. I find the fruits and vegetables lining the walls as are the milk, cheeses, and yogurts plus meats, chicken, and fish. Everything is on the circumference of the store without my tempting fate by going down difficult aisles that feel like a minefield. I avoided these areas for years.

But…I must warn you, some stores are on to us "healthy eaters" and they've moved around the foods, forcing us to enter the combat zone in order to reach our clean foods. Or I'll be snagging some nice veggies and fruits, and right in front of me, I'll see donuts and snack cakes dangling out of an end cap on a side aisle.

Keep focused on what you need and nothing else, and you'll be just fine. Remember you're investing in you—self-love and self-care. Your body is your temple, a gift from *your* Divine Source.

Now, regardless of where I am, I can buy what I need. One year in California, I walked to the local store, carrying back several bags to my hotel room where I was attending a conference. I had a small fridge and microwave in the room, which I requested for medicinal purposes—hence the charge was waived. Food is medicine.

I was set. I had picked up a roasted chicken, salad fixings, fresh fruit, and yogurt, along with a few sweet and white potatoes, and olive oil. I'd made my own muffins at home and packed those, knowing they would be my breakfast. Easy-schmeezy. I had nothing to want for.

A Work in Progress

Picking out food to eat wasn't always so easy for me. We are all works in progress. One year, at the beginning of my quest, I attended a conference in Tennessee, where I requested a room with a view. I luxuriated in a queen-sized bed overlooking a nice view of a harbor with boats bobbing up and down. I had also requested a room with a full bath, an extravagance I take advantage of on every trip. I was set.

I unpacked my foods, as I had stopped at the grocery store before checking in. ensuring I had all that I needed for a successful weekend. I stretched out on the bed with a good book as I could enjoy a few hours before going to the first event. In the stillness I heard this *click, hum, and click, click, click*...and looked up and saw another fridge I hadn't noticed at first. It had red lights swirling all around as if it were a Las Vegas gambling machine, beckoning me to come closer. I squinted to get a better look and to my shock saw that it was fully stocked with liquor, beers, soda pops and candy bars. Eureka!!

My heart began to pound, and worry overtook me. I was afraid I'd cave. But I pushed such thoughts out of my mind, as I had things to do to prepare for the sessions. Out and about, I attended the first event, and then the second, and then third, not giving the red flashing lights another thought. In between morning and evening sessions I made my way back to my room for my prepared lunch, again not even thinking about the loaded fridge.

Later that evening, after a lovely dinner with the other attendees, I returned to my room with a full belly, and a happy heart. I'd learned a lot, and I felt good. I pushed away whatever concerns I'd had earlier that day. I was strong, and would be just fine. I took a long, hot bath and felt great as I crawled into bed, exhausted from a long day of talks.

As I was drifting off to sleep, the red lights kept swirling round and round as if to say, *Come here. I've got goodies for you to eat.* I jumped out of bed, pulling the extra quilt in the closet over the fridge, where it stayed the rest of the event.

Once back in bed I felt fine…safe, drifting off to never-never land, until I heard a knock on my door, which I ignored, hoping it would go away. **Knock, knock, knock.** *"Hello, it's the midnight madness snack attack tray…heloooooo!"* What!

I opened the door to a widely smiling Asian girl, velvet black hair cascading down her back, and with steel-blue eyes, beckoning me to come closer as she stood there with a cord around her neck to balance the tray she was carrying—a tray filled with *every* decadent chocolate treat you can imagine. I wanted to dive in and become a part of that tray. *I didn't.* I declined and closed the door in complete awe of what had just transpired.

Test one, the flashing fridge, and now test two, a tray full of pure heaven, both behind me. I was ready for anything else. Bring it on.

I made it through, and now look back fondly at those earlier times. Food doesn't make the event. The event makes the event. I don't recall one food I've eaten at any of the conferences I've been to, and I've been to many, but I do hold close the forever treasured lectures, information, and long-term friendships I embedded within.

Vigilance Goes a Long Way

The same can happen for you too. Before you arrive at your destination, pack the foods you can transport, learn what restaurants are nearby, and gather up menus, as most are posted online these days. Ask the hotel to provide a microwave and fridge, as most will. Learn where the closest grocery stores are located to stock the foods you'll need between restaurant stops, and you're sure to be good to go. If you make up your mind to succeed, you will—but if you leave room for the maybe, you won't.

You'll feel fabulous fueling with real foods. You'll be able *to think well, love well, and sleep well, if you've dined well.* I'm positive.

I'm certain if you have children, you pack snacks for them. Why? Because you want to be prepared for the moment they cry for food, and/or a drink. And surely they will. Do the same for yourself. Pack your foods and drinks…

Ahhh, Italia

On our first night in Vicenza, Italy, a few years back, I, my sister Mickey, and her family, made our way to the local grocery store, not speaking the language, and not knowing the store set-up, where most of the foods were. But food is food the whole world 'round, and eventually we figured out where the fresh foods were, and snagged all that we needed.

The food was more expensive then in the States, and meats seemed harder to come by, but we managed. We were prepared with a list of needs, not wants, and made the food question work. Our meals were magical, as we dined outside on the terrace, overlooking a backdrop of mountains. The trip was totally amazing, as I describe in other chapters, but our remaining vigilant reinforced the reality that you can travel and stay on course with healthy living and lifestyle strategies.

Our little group focused on hiking and walking, and simply being family. I don't recall the foods so much as I do the company. And that's just the point. Eating is a lovely activity, and certainly a necessity for life, but it is not the event. The event is who you're eating with.

And Then There's Morris

Take Morris, a lovely English chap, who drives a semi-rig cross-country, delivering highly secured cargo from one end of the US to the other. Morris has been everywhere and has eaten in many truck stops, and out at fine dinning too. Once upon a time Morris was hefting an extra two-hundred pounds. He blamed it on his job, saying he *had* to eat what was available to him while on the road—that in no realistic way could he eat clean and healthy.

I listened.

Morris had carried extra weight his entire life, as far back as he could remember after moving to the US. He had been born and raised in a small town in England—Dedham, Essex, England—which he believed to be the most beautiful village in all of this country. He loved fishing with his grandpa at the river that flowed through his quaint town.

"Life was good—really, really good—in this town filled with charm," said Morris as he was transported via his deeply etched memory to where the air was crisp and fresh with rolling hills reflecting a faint, intermittent glow around him in lush green foliage, and cozy little cottages scattered about.

Morris looked off into the distance as he recounted the fishing stories as the best time in all of his life, in the charming three-room cottage with his beloved grandpa, warmed by the fireplace, burning the wood and brush Morris had gathered. After a lovely fish fry, they'd rest by the fire, faces flushed from the heat, and Grandpa would talk of his adventures, with Morris hanging onto each and every word that fell from Grandpa's lips.

Life changed when circumstances yanked Morris away from England to New York City for a few years, before he landed in South Florida, where he began to pile on the excess weight. After earning a degree in business, Morris started his trucking business, buying a sleek rig he named Bessie to live a life he'd dreamt of since he was a child. Morris loved to travel in his rig through small towns, up and down the winding roads to interesting stops along the way. He was a free spirit.

Morris was a happy guy who was searching for England in every quaint town he passed through, dropping off this and that load of precious cargo. He loved the little restaurants, small-town charm, and the locals—all of which transported him back to the beloved, quaint little town that once was.

As we began our work together unpacking where his eating frenzy began, Morris began to have an awareness that he was trying to recreate a time that was so magical in his life. The more we explored his memories, the more evident became the sense that the food wasn't what filled his heart, the key was the memories of the people he had loved.

We began to design ways he could continue to enjoy his perfect job without jeopardizing his health. As we dove into the *Come Shop with Me* discussion, Morris started to understand how to work his way through a grocery store without being derailed by the junk-food aisles. At first, he was resistant about even going into the grocery stores while out on the road. Ingrained in his psyche was that work and travel involved fast food stops, and he dragged along junk foods that were easy to eat while driving.

We knocked off one challenge after the other until we carved out a healthy lifestyle for him both on the road and off. Morris first joined Planet Fitness, one of the largest and most affordable national fitness centers, which over the years has spread to just about every state in the country, certainly those that Morris and Bessie pass through. Morris then began to stock a small refrigerated cooler in his rig with fresh fruits, lean meats, raw and cooked veggies, and good sources of fats, along with unprocessed starches.

Morris made sure to eat his meals every four to five hours to avoid too much hunger, and long before leaving his home state learned where the best restaurants were located on his routes. The hotels he stayed at quickly discovered that Morris expected a microwave and small fridge in the room. He made a home away from home, whether in his rig, hotel, restaurant, or fitness center, working in his expected daily routine.

Morris permitted himself no such thing as an off-day from living right. All days were healthy eating days for him, whether he was far from home, home, or in another country. *His food was his food, and everything else was not.* Morris began to live his best life.

To date, Morris is at the right weight for his body size and age. He feels strong and confident that he is now living life on purpose. He loves his work and home life. As he saved money eating out less and making better money choices, he was able to squirrel away enough to afford one of those quaint little cottages in England. Now he can escape there several times of year when his place isn't rented out as an Airbnb, earning money while he's on the road. He's made the best of all worlds, traveling, working, and enjoying his home life, to meet all his dreams.

Okay, so now you understand the importance of working your foods, no matter where you are, by finding a grocery market, leaving little risk of sabotaging your healthy efforts. So what next? What about how to cook these lovely foods (Chapter 16) in a way that's enjoyable?

Personal Inventory Questions

1. Do you make excuses why you need to eat this or that during a hotel outing? What reasons might be behind this, such as a memory connection?
2. What memory of temptation comes to mind on one of your excursions, business or pleasure? Review the memory, and imagine what you could do differently. Often these memories fuel our next experience, but now you're

breaking the habit, moving into new territory—creating a new beginning going forward.

3. Do you pack foods in preparation for a trip? And if so, what foods are you inclined to bring? Are they healthy, or something you just take with because, well that's just what you do. If the reason is the latter, consider revamping your food list to create your new norm.
4. Do you think well, love well, and sleep well? Are you living your life on purpose? Do you feel how you think, love, and sleep connects to whether or not you dine well? What's your dream life, and how close to it are you?
5. Have you ever gone to a fitness center or gym outside of your place of living? Does doing such a thing seem feasible? Perhaps you're shy and feel uncomfortable in a new environment. Consider that most of the people in the fitness center attached to the hotel, if not all, are new customers too. And if the fitness gym is a franchise, it will most likely be set up like the gym in your own town, and not feel so foreign, after all.
6. How do you relate to Morris? Was your childhood shaken up in some way that your food, and weight, became an issue for you? We tend to be caught up in what was imprinted during our earlier years, but that doesn't need to make up who you are in your latter years. You have the power to make that shift.
7. Often money becomes the excuse for not living our best life possible. How does money play into your health routine, in a good way or bad?
8. Have you ever had your best health plans ruined due to unexpected situations in a hotel room stocked with candies, chips, and alcohol? If so, what was the outcome? How can you rewrite the script?
9. If you had to pinpoint one area in this chapter that really resonated with you, what would it be, and how would you

work an idea sparked by it into your life in a positive manner?

10. Do you bring your foods with you when you travel? If you do, are they healthy-choice foods, or junk foods that you think you ***need*** to eat in order to have a good stay? Why or why not is that the case?

Chapter 16

Come Cook with Me

Acknowledging the good
that you already have in your life
is the foundation for all abundance.
~Eckhart Tolle

What type of abundance do you wish for? Money, material possessions, or perhaps spiritual awareness in your life? What about acknowledging what you already have. Often we're searching for something that's right in front of us. What you want may not be *out there*, but rather in you.

You don't need a village in order to jump on board with your cooking, but instead you have to take responsibility for yourself. You can play the blame game, or make excuses as to why you have to eat this or that, but really, making a food plan is quite simple. You don't have to buy every new diet book that hits the shelves with ***the*** diet that works. I'm here to tell you some "special" way of eating in order to live well doesn't exist. Food is food, and here in America we're blessed with a plenitude of it. All that's needed is for you to choose the right foods and assemble them in a way that's enticing, nutritious, and delicious to you.

The best means to conquer food challenges and create a healthy relationship with each meal is to design meals that work for *you*. My ideas are only suggestions—and not etched in stone. If you bend the menu to fit your ideal way of eating, you'll be on your way to a healthy practice of connecting to food, *always*. No longer will your diet be based in an on-and-off, good-and-bad mentality, but rather your food is your food, and everything else is not.

Once you establish and launch your way of eating, regardless of where you are, or who you're with, you'll begin to experience true freedom in your relationship with food, your body, and your overall life.

Mastering the Chef in You

In the previous chapter I highlighted shopping for foods, and in the chapter to come, we'll talk about the sacred art of mealtime and sharing conversations and stories of the day and times, but for now, let's talk about actually cooking foods. Some people, maybe even you, have a knack for whipping up lovely meals, while others rely on a freezer-to-microwave kind of cooking. (I'm somewhere in between the two.)

Cooking provides you with an opportunity to detach from your phone and television, and instead connect to the richness of the moment. You now have a chance to be present and one with the food you're about to prepare. Over the years I've delved into the practice of present living, and linking with my Higher Source, or the Universe, or the Divine, or God—whatever you chose to call your *connection*. You can do this, too, as you begin to fix your meal.

The art of cooking is a basic skill that can turn a meal into a miraculous concoction fabricated from love and motivated expression. Meal preparation time provides a space for you to discover your signature—your legacy—that you will pass down for generations to come.

One way to build your bequest is to orchestrate rituals of nurturing the body with earthly foods—God's foods. Maybe in childhood Mom simmered her famous chicken soup using vegetables from the garden, or Grandma served *incredible* homemade applesauce made from apples off the tree in the yard. These were spiritual moments of inspiration, shared meals constructed with affection for those around the table.

Please understand up front, I'm no Martha Stewart—or Julia Childs, for those of you who grew up with her singing on television in the makeshift kitchen, all while cooking and sipping wine, toasting to all the would-be chefs of America. No, I'm definitely not one of those. They are/were amazing cooks, and my mother was too. Mom could put together a topnotch meal at a moment's notice. Somehow, I didn't inherit her cooking genes. But what I have learned to do is to come up with palatable foods in abundance that are delicious, clean, and affordable.

Keep in mind no laws reign around spirituality and bringing creative meals to your table, whether the meal is for you alone, or for a large group.

The Magic of Apple, Polenta, and Tofu

One of my favorite foods to share with loved ones and to make on long weekends is my famous Breakfast Apple-Polenta-Tofu Delight. They are easy to make, and transport. I prepare and pack several breakfast servings, to take the *think* out of what to eat. If you start the day right, your chances to finish on a healthy course are pretty darn good.

When making this tofu delight, you can use a fruit of your choice, but I prefer a chopped apple, plus 1 cup cooked corn grits in cubes (cook according to the package and pour into flat container to cool, then cut in cubes), liquid sweetener to taste (optional), vanilla, cinnamon, ginger, and/or nutmeg to taste, 6 ounces firm tofu, cubed, 1 teaspoon coconut oil.

Brown firm tofu in pan with spices—then add and brown the remaining ingredients, corn grits and margarine. Stir until brown then add sweetener to grits. Once browned, fold in the apples and cook a few minutes—I like mine crispy so I cook this a little longer than you might. Place all ingredients in a bowl and top with two tablespoons of fat-free plain yogurt or Greek yogurt if you want it thicker and creamier.

Fruity Pancakes

I also find that pancakes make a lovely breakfast in the morning, using half a cup of oat bran, one cup of raspberries and bananas, a tablespoon of straight dark cocoa, one teaspoon of real vanilla, and two eggs, with a pinch of salt and cinnamon. Mix well, form into three pancakes that you'll pan cook, flipping them once they're browned on one side. Top with a few tablespoons of fat-free Greek yogurt, and you have an amazing, satisfying breakfast. These too will freeze nicely, and can be brought along on trips. Again, I change up the fruits for variety.

Leftovers

Another absolute favorite breakfast of mine starts by working with leftovers from the night before. One particular choice that comes to mind is based on cutting four ounces of leftover steak into large cubes, browning that with mushrooms and onions, while in the oven under the broiler placing six ounces of leftover sweet potatoes sliced in wedges topped with cinnamon, sea salt, and coconut oil. Leave in till browned and crispy. Once all is cooked, I line my plate with steak covered in mushrooms and onions, sweet potato browned to perfection, and slices of ripe cantaloupe. On the table I provide tea with almond milk, and I'm feeling mighty happy.

A Little Salmon Anyone?

Salmon is a staple in my home. I purchase a large slab from Sam's Club … brush with mustard and bay spice, then broil for twenty-six minutes. The fish comes out golden brown and totally delicious. I serve with brown rice, a spring lettuce mix and spinach salad with tomatoes, avocado, onion, and romaine, topped with olive oil and vinegar. This is a very easy meal, taking under thirty minutes to make, with tons of leftovers to bring with you when you travel or have a getaway weekend. The salmon is delicious cold on a bed of lettuce or served with asparagus spears.

Cooking as an art, rather than a chore, turns your foods into an experience, a banquet of healing from the inside out. Cooking is very spiritual, not just the way you cook, but also the intention with which you do it. Too often, we convince ourselves that cooking a meal is too hard, too time consuming, too expensive, or simply boring, but it's not.

This isn't to say going out to eat is a bad thing—for surely it's not. But sharing a meal with the family cooked from foods you picked from the garden, or even chose at the supermarket, makes the experience a convivial one, a way of connecting to others. Entering your home with the aroma of fresh stew coming from the crock pot warms the heart, bringing a feeling of family together and love.

Christy's 7-Layer Incredible Salad

I've heard people say that food is always so much better when someone you love cooks it for you. *Your* Uncle Lou's famous grilled chicken with his secret spices, or Aunt Jenny's famous cod, or my sister Christy's INCREDIBLE seven-layer salad, with a layer of romaine lettuce, followed by a layer of avocado, and then a layer of peas, and a layer of mushrooms—and between each layer a mayonnaise dressing—a combo that was a little taste of heaven. This salad was a meal in and of itself.

Some of my fondest memories are of watching my mother slicing mushrooms and onions and celery for whatever blend she was cooking up. And then smelling it for hours on end as it cooked, knowing that soon we'd gather and eat. We didn't join daily for family meals, so when we did, the occasion was marked in my mind as one of the most delightful parts of my childhood.

Think back to your food memories and how you felt. Perhaps your memories are truly wonderful, or maybe not so good. In either situation, you have the ability to create the aroma you want in your home. You have the power to make more memories to pass down for generations to come.

Recreate Your Kitchen Space

The kitchen once was thought of as a sacred place, and now it's almost a foreign area for many, only equipped with a microwave and fast foods. If you want more abundance financially, emotionally, and spiritually, start with your kitchen, carving out a space that speaks to you so you can begin to create cost-effective, homemade meals. Self-care begins with preparing foods because you're worth it.

Maybe your kitchen doesn't feel right; if so, change it. Clear off the counters and put some flowers or pretty ceramic bowls or cups there. When I was in Italy, I bought a lovely handmade china platter with blue flowers framing the border to rest my cooking spoon on, along with a deep yellow and purple pitcher, and a large spoon of the same colors. I placed the plate on my counter as an ever reminder of my trip, and to make my kitchen sing with joy. You might find canisters or jars or some other unique pieces to make this spot your signature kitchen—a place where you want to sit and sip your coffee or tea, and take it all in.

The kitchen is the heart of the home, the gathering place for family, friends, and acquaintances. It's the place to build memories around laughter, tears, and maybe even shouts of joy—or not. It's that place for all happenings. Your food festivities can start with a personal meal, a family meal, or an out-and-out party—all from the heart of your home.

Often I hear, "I'm alone, so why should I cook?" I say, because you're worth it. Cooking for yourself is a message of love. And buying and cooking your own food saves hundreds of dollars a year—money you can use for your next trip.

Break the chain of the SAD—Standard American Diet—and base your menu on a healthy way of eating, rather than consuming high-fat, processed foods.

Keep the cooking simple. When you prepare a meal, have your staples on hand, as suggested in Chapter 15—Come Shop with Me! Foods on hand make preparation, and commitment, much more likely.

Grilling on the weekends, when you have get-togethers, is an easy way to stay on point with your eating plan. A favorite in our household is hamburgers stuffed with Portobello mushrooms, peppers, onions, and shaved parmesan cheese served with skewers of peppers and sweet potatoes, and roasted green beans marinated in garlic, lemon, and olive oil, and sprinkled with Himalayan pink sea salt. Easy, delicious, and practically zero clean up.

Another choice of ours is spicy chicken breasts with air-fried sweet potatoes and fresh asparagus topped by drizzled olive oil. Simply lay out your chicken breasts in a foil-lined roasting pan. Top with Pace brand salsa or any salsa you prefer that isn't laced with sugar. Include fresh garlic and sea salt. Bake at 400 for two hours, then let sit for thirty minutes. The sauce will caramelize, making an incredible eating experience. The sweet potatoes are tossed in no more than a tablespoon of olive oil and spicy seasoning and air fried for the allotted time your air frying device indicates. Plate the above alongside roasted asparagus with chunks of mushrooms cooked at a lower level in the oven after one hour of the chicken cooking.

Don't let your crock pot be a stranger. It can be cooking for you while you're swimming in the pool, walking along the ocean, hiking in the fields, sailing in the sea, or whatever it is you do on the weekends and vacations. A favorite of mine is to take an entire roast beef, cutting it in two to fit in the crock pot, then adding onions, garlic, and spices and letting it slow cook for the entire day after one hour on high. Add brown rice to your rice cooker plus steamed vegetables of your choice, and voila you have a wonderful meal that makes for great leftovers.

If you're a Martha Stewart type, even better, as you'll be able to take these very simple recipes and raise them up to something spectacular. Cooking is an art and quite relaxing if you don't fight it—lean in and let the magic happen.

You might be asking how much food to eat. Good question. I'm a food addict/exercise bulimic in recovery. To arrive at the place I'm at now, I did weigh and measure my food for years to keep the portions right. I tended to go too little, or when bingeing, too much. You have to decide for yourself if you need to weigh and measure, which I talk about at great length in my first book, *Release Your Obsession with Food: Heal from the Inside Out.* I also have an entire chapter of recipes there that you might find of interest.

To date, I only weigh and measure my foods at home, but not in front of people other than my family. I don't want to be the center of conversation or up for display, but in private I do measure to keep myself on point. I was never one to bring scales and measuring aids with me to restaurants, but you can if you're comfortable with that. I was always able to eyeball the food to measure. Now my food observations are so honed that I automatically stop when I've eaten the right amount. To be overfull or under isn't comfortable for me.

Be inventive and you'll find cooking easy, fun, and a way to move the sacred meal into reality rather than just being an idea. ***Acknowledging the good that you already have in your life is the foundation for all abundance*** as Mr. Tolle says.

Creating meals with intention goes a long way—it's your legacy. Every food you prepare with heart brings a connection, and an opportunity to pay it forward. Give thanks and praise for what you have.

Now take what you know and move forward to anywhere in the world and share meals that are whole and real and weave more memories to pass down to your loved ones as you'll see in Chapter 17: The Sacred Art of Mealtime.

Personal Inventory Questions

1. What type of abundance do you wish for? Money, material possessions or spiritual awareness? What about acknowledging what you already have?
2. Often we're searching for something that's right in front of us all along. What are you searching for?
3. The best way to conquer food challenges and assure a healthy relationship with each meal is to design meals that work for you. My ideas are only suggestions—and not etched in stone. What foods fit you and your lifestyle?
4. What can you do to change the way you relate to foods in your home—in your kitchen?
5. Cooking and preparing meals is not only a people connection but a spiritual one as well. It provides an opportunity to disconnect from your phone and television, and instead connect to the richness of the moment. What would eating unplugged from electronics be like for you?
6. What would building a spiritual practice around food look like for you?

7. One of my favorite foods to share with loved ones and to carry with me when traveling are homemade muffins. They're easy to make, freeze, and transport. What food can you share with others and transport as well when traveling?
8. The kitchen is the heart of the home. It's the gathering place for family, friends, and acquaintances. How have you made your kitchen the heart of your home?
   Don't let your crock pot be a stranger. What creative foods can you prepare for your next gathering?
9. Many influential television personalities formed my opinion of cooking. Who made an impression on you? What parts of cooking food do you work into your healthy eating lifestyle?
10. Many influential television personalities formed my opinion of cooking. Who made an impression on you? What parts of cooking food do you work into your healthy eating lifestyle?

Chapter 17

The Sacred Art of Mealtime

I want to be remembered
as a person who wanted to be free…
so other people would be also free.
~Rosa Parks

The theme of this book is how to become free with your food so that you can be free with your food. Kind of a twist on words, but once you glean an understanding of food and how to make peace with it, you will truly become free to enjoy a wide array of real foods.

Rosa Parks' words are powerful ones that we can all learn from and in individual ways adopt. She opened doors for many women and for the African American population—and for you too, whatever ethnicity you claim. Rosa was brave and pushed past all the naysayers and dived into turbulent and most feared waters.

You can ignore all the naysayers too, and move through circumstances you most fear, also, with a sense of peace and while asserting your authentic personhood. Who are these naysayers, you might ask? Well, the ones who say it's not realistic for you to choose a peach instead of a luscious-looking piece of chocolate cake. Let's ponder.

What Is Realistic?

What is realistic? The dictionary powered by Oxford Dictionaries, for one thing defines *realistic* as "having or showing a sensible and practical idea of what can be achieved or expected." Realistic is also "representing familiar things in a way that is accurate or true to life."

Okay, is it familiar/true to life to eat cake when others are eating such a sweet treat? Yes, of course. But is getting a headache, shakes, and an uncontrollable desire to eat the entire cake, along with anything and everything else that is in front of you, also familiar/true to life? Yes, for sure—these symptoms are familiar and true to life for the compulsive eater, eating addict, food addict, and those described by any other phrase who can't control their food intake, especially if indulging in sugar, flour, and/or wheat.

So the naysayers aren't showing a sensible and practical idea of what can be achieved or expected when they say such things as, "Have a bite. It won't hurt you." Or "Just this once." Or, "Not eating cake isn't realistic." These folks aren't in your head—only you are. And only *you* can understand the devastation and destruction one supposedly innocent piece of cake can cause you.

With that bite, the road less traveled will become total mayhem.

Meals are to be sacred, and if you're in a tizzy, the meal isn't so sacred. So take heed of Ms. Rosa Parks, and grab your freedom. Your freedom in this case will be from your cheat-day mentality.

Rosa Louise McCauley Parks was an American activist in the civil rights movement. She is best remembered for her pivotal role in the Montgomery bus boycott. Known as the "first lady of civil rights" and "the mother of the freedom movement," Ms. Parks took a brave stand when she refused to surrender her seat to a white passenger on a segregated bus in Montgomery, Alabama, catapulting the nation into a popular effort to end racial segregation of public facilities.

Ms. Parks is remembered as a person who wanted to be free so that other people could also be free.

I began my quest to free those with food addictions from obsessing over and indulging in (whatever kind of) foods when I was in my thirties, as I tried to understand why the food grip was so tight on me. I wanted to figure out what was going on with me so that I also could figure out what was happening with others. One of the first realizations I had was that most families were no longer sharing meals together.

I must admit I didn't figure this out on my own because at the time I was knee deep in my binge eating disorder and bulimia through exercise. I was focused solely on how skinny I needed to be rather than how healthy I should be. I wasn't able to see things that were happening as they really were, or understand how to deal with them in a practical way.

I only looked at what I wanted or hoped for—which was to eat whatever I desired, be in control of my food intake, and live in a skinny body. This wasn't realistic, given my food addiction, hypoglycemia, and bulimia. I was a hot mess and tried to bend the situation to my will rather step into a sensible, appropriate (realistic) way to handle my health.

After the birth of my son, I fell into the habit of eating my meal separately from him. He had the baby meal, and I was glued to the TV with the big person's meal. At the time we had a coffee table where we'd plop on the floor with our goodies and chow down.

Long after my boy was in bed, I continued gulping and inhaling foods while watching *The Tonight Show* with Johnny

Carson, eating a tremendous amount of sugary, flour-laced foods in private—which food addicts tend to do.

Food addicts don't want to be seen eating as they slip into a coma-like state of existence, eating an enormous amount of food voraciously in a brief amount of time, oblivious to their "full" signal.

My current husband, then boyfriend, visited our little family on many evenings when my son was about to turn four. Once he discovered how we were eating our meals, he was appalled. He wanted us to sit *at a table* with plates set out nicely, forks, knives, and spoons carefully placed on napkins with a nice centerpiece to make the meal an event.

What! I was a tad annoyed, and Benjamin was full-blown angry. He didn't like *"that man"* telling us we needed to eat at a table. I really didn't want to rearrange our routine, either. But two years later, "that man" and I were married, living in a new home, eating meals together as a family *at the table.*

Now this may seem like basic 101 to you, but I assure you such an arrangement was not familiar to me. From my recollection, my mother only called for mealtime as a family on Sundays, when we'd all gather together for breakfast, lunch, and dinner. Other than that, food time meant TV dinners and the television.

This is not to say my family of origin never ever had mealtime together because I assure you we did, but certainly not as often as other families in the neighborhood, which was my only barometer at that period. But the times we did gather as a family were truly amazing—and sacred. I have many, many fond memories of those Sunday meals, and meals with my great-grandma Baba, up at our summer home in Wisconsin. Those meals were pure heaven. We laughed and listened to the funny stories Mom, Grandma Ruth, and Great-grandma Baba shared.

I loved having time as a family, but somehow that was lost during everyday life when we were going to school during the workweek. I do recall saying my prayers before a meal at school and often with the family when we were little, but somehow that was forgotten or slipped into the ether.

When we discovered McDonald's, their takeout became a big food event…eating at the coffee table on the floor, sprawled out watching *Bonanza* or *The Ed Sullivan Show* among others. These are fond memories, for sure, but not of us as a family talking and sharing the day's events. So I carried on this same tradition with my toddler, passing down my experience eating at the coffee table—a trend that could have gone on, but thank goodness we soon stopped.

Joining at the Table

My husband's insistence that we share meals at the table was the beginning of the Sacred Art of Mealtime for me, which has continued since. Laughter, stories, serious conversations took place at the table, night after night, impressing on our two sons how important meals and family were. Not only do family meals connect family, but also they build memories for a lifetime.

Transforming the seemingly mundane into service to yourself and others, into fulfillment, into a spiritual practice bathed in love can be a sacred experience for you in a very personal way.

You can light candles of lovely scents that will blend well with eating, lower the lights, and/or open the windows to let in the fresh air. You can put on soft music or loud rock and roll—whatever feeds your heart, your soul. Feel free to create a ceremony filled with joy as you power through tasks that might have once seemed more like chores.

Julie Penkalski in her "The Importance of Family Mealtime" (retrieved from the Family & Children's Center blog) notes that family meals tend to be more nutritious than casually eaten solitary meals, based on a Harvard study that found families who eat together are twice as likely to eat their five servings of fruits and vegetables as families than those who don't eat jointly. Better yet, studies found that kids who eat family meals most often eat a wider variety of foods and become less picky eaters.

Families who eat together simply tend to be healthier and happier because they not only eat together, they talk together, and make mealtime a family time. We started the process of family time early in our sons' lives, reaping the rewards today. Gathering for a meal wasn't a maybe, it was a must. The family cooperated in setting the table and cleaning up afterward. The television was off and soft music on.

Family Gathering Tips:

1. Make meals a joint event by inviting family members' input into upcoming meals at the dinner table, so all feel involved and look forward to the next family meal gathering.
2. Prepare meals together as a family. One member can set the table, while another might assist in the cooking preparation.
3. Don't allow one person to eat different foods than the others—all meals are best shared. Often families make the mistake of separating foods, where one eats one meal and others another. When all eat the same foods, this not only builds a more communal family but also avoids creating the "picky eater." Where medical necessity mandates one family member must or can't eat a certain food, that food can still be presented on the table for all.
4. Make food presentable—a visual presentation is inviting. Kids aren't always fond of fish, vegetables, or other "healthy" foods, but if you offer foods in a delightful arrangement they become more palatable. For example, a

red tomato sauce can harbor and hide loads of vegetables without a child detecting their presence.

5. Don't talk about family meals, just have them. Too often, the household agrees they're going to start sharing meals as a family, but they never begin. Take action rather than talking without follow-through.
6. Take turns cooking a scheduled meal. For instance, you make the meal one night, your husband another, and the kids another—allowing variety and permitting control to be surrendered to different family members.
7. Cleanup shouldn't be the cook's responsibility, but rather a family joint-effort affair. Cleanups are faster when cooperative and can actually be loads of fun as the conversation continues along with family bonding. You're teaching the art of cleanup not as a chore but as a fun event. The entire meal from preparation, to feasting, to cleaning up becomes the art of the meal.
8. If the thought of family dinners is daunting, begin with a family breakfast, brunch, or lunch to start the ball rolling. In time, the consistency of at least one meal together each day becomes the norm—and an expectation.
9. Creating meals as a unit is less expensive than eating out, ordering takeout, or eating boxed foods. Make shopping for lovely foods at the grocery store a group occasion rather than having one person making all the choices.
10. Foods that are cooked from scratch are fresh, meaning more nutritious, and for sure, can be managed without sugar, poor quality fats, or too much sodium, because you're controlling what's going into the meal preparation.

Study after study shows mealtime is a powerful occasion for blending and mending families. When the family dinner is created with love and unity, it doesn't have to be viewed as a burdensome chore, especially after a long work and/or school day.

The benefits of family dinners are beyond the scope of this chapter—in fact such a conversation could fuel an entire book. But just to scratch the surface, family mealtime is shown to teach unity, love, and family connectedness. Families joined in this fundamental way tend to have higher self-esteem, greater sense of resilience, lower risk of substance abuse, and yes, even lower risk of teen pregnancy.

How something so basic as mealtime can lead to such great successes seems almost too good to be true. Try it—you might just like the results when you practice the art of family mealtime.

Think of Rosa Parks as she braved her way into foreign territory, uniting people of all sorts. You, too, can be remembered as a person who wanted to be free and to free others from their food challenges and their fragmented families—simply by sharing a meal.

Now that you're armed and ready for jumping into the sacred art of family meals, let's turn to Chapter 18 and make every day a good day as we pull the food festivity together.

Personal Inventory Questions

1. Throughout this book, the theme focuses on becoming free with your food so that you can be free with your food. Do you make excuses for why you need to eat this or that during family meals?
2. Rosa Parks was brave, standing up under volatile conditions for women's rights and for the African American population. Although food choices may not seem such an explosive issue, society often mocks those who choose to eat clean and healthy, abstaining from processed foods. How do you process this?

3. You can push past all the naysayers too, and move through feared and turbulent times, holding the space for peace and authenticity. Who are your naysayers?
4. Is choosing real foods from the ground, trees, sky, and seas realistic?
5. When was the last time your family ate together? After reading this chapter, what can you learn from your recent meal experience?
6. Sometimes when we are hyper-focused on our personal food challenges, we miss what's happening with the family dynamics food-wise. Are you fixated on how skinny you *need* to be rather than how healthy you want to be?
7. After the birth of my first son, I slipped into the habit of eating separate meals. He had the baby meal, and I was glued to the TV with the big person's meal. Take a moment to assess how your family meals came together, and come together.
8. Did fast foods change the trajectory of your family mealtime as a child?
9. After reading the section on family mealtime tips, what ideas can you pull together for your family dynamic?
10. Ms. Parks is remembered as a person who wanted to be free so that other people could also be free. Wouldn't you too like to be free from your cheat days and processed foods and share a new way of family mealtime to pass down to your children? When was the last time you shared a meal united with your loved ones?

Chapter 18

Every Day a Good Day

Take the first step, and your mind
will mobilize all its forces to your aid.
But the first essential is that you begin.
Once the battle is started,
all that is within and without you
will come to your assistance.
~Robert Collier

Every day is a new opportunity to make the day a good one, no matter what happened yesterday, last week, last year, or a lifetime ago. Every day is a good day, no matter where you are: London, Italy, France, Tennessee, or at home for a long weekend.

This is not to say you won't have a bad day now and again, for surely you will, but every day of life is an opportunity for change. We've all had those days when we wish the day wasn't—but do we really want this? No, we wish we felt better, or that our day were unfolding more enjoyably.

Perhaps we wish for tomorrow, or that vacation, or a long weekend, or we remember a better yesterday, or last year, or *when we were younger*. But is that wish really for tomorrow—or for better times? Maybe our discomfort isn't about tomorrow or yesterday, but rather springs from fear—a distressing emotion aroused by impending, imagined angst, or more specifically the worry about the unknown—a disquiet over some future event you may dread. But the feared-of moment isn't here, so it's not real. All we have is today, or more specifically, this moment. We have now. And you have the opportunity to make ***now*** your very best time ever.

Take the first step, and your mind will mobilize all its forces to your aid. Ah, but you might say, how can I take the first step when I'm so tired, when my mind is bogged down with the weight of life? All that's required is that first try, and much can change.

Maxi's Journey

Not long ago, a patient, I'll call her Maxi, texted me to tell me she wasn't doing so great. That she was feeling really sad and anxious, for no apparent reason.

Of course I began my usual series of questions such as: "Are you taking your medications? Did something happen? Are you alone? Who can you call for support?" Maxi was once a bubbly, blue-eyed blonde with an infectious smile that had become foreign to her. Family and friends were starting to notice her poor mood and make comments. Nothing was worthwhile to her any longer, it seemed. She only saw doom and gloom ahead. The laughter and the spark were gone.

Maxi had just returned from a lovely vacation in Southern California where she'd spent time with her two best childhood friends. She'd talked and dreamed of this trip for months, but when she arrived, she was filled with anxiety and fear. Fear of what the three were going to do. Fear of whether she'd have enough to eat. Fear that she'd eat too much. Fear she'd not eat enough. Fear that her clothes wouldn't fit. Fear of not having the energy to keep up with her girlfriends, or if she'd need a nap and not be able to fit one in.

Maxi was gripped by fear, yet she'd been planning and dreaming about this trip for months. In fact, everything Maxi feared came to fruition. She had a miserable trip. Why? Well, perhaps Maxi didn't *take the first step;* hence, her mind was unable to mobilize all its forces to her aid. *But the first essential is that you begin*…and Maxi wasn't able to. *Once the battle is started, all that is within and without you will come to your assistance.*

You see the first essential is that you begin. Maxi didn't begin. She believed in the fears that gripped her so tightly that they *became* her experience. She had "old talk" murmuring, talk she'd been carrying around her entire life.

This internal commentary about her body and presentation drove her self-doubt. And spending time with childhood friends in an area where she grew up only strengthened her feeling of doom and gloom. Memories of the not-so-good times came flooding in. This magical vacation she'd dreamt about for months on end turned into a painful emotional experience. She entertained childhood memories of not fitting in, not being good enough, and worse…*being too fat.*

Once the battle is started, all that is within and without you will come to your assistance. But if you never start, or if you start with the wrong message, then what will come to your assistance will only be negative self-talk of shame, blame, and judging yourself.

Society reinforces that we are what we look like. Certain expectations are put in front of us day in and day out. So on this lovely trip, rather than working with the mantra *Every day is a good day*, Maxi was working with the internal dialogue of *I'm not good enough, thin enough, pretty enough, or smart enough*, all of which clouded her "good day" approach.

And to make matters worse, Maxi's two girlfriends were that "perfect picture" sort society sets as a standard, a level that most of us can't attain. They both were tall and thin, with long, flowing hair, one having locks of golden hues with perfect curls, and the other enjoying auburn and straight tresses tumbling down to the middle of her back. The young women were both quick to laugh and joke and share stories of their love lives and jobs that they prospered in.

As for Maxi, she felt trapped in her job with no room to move up, no love life at all, and nothing to look forward to. All she had to count on were memories of her father saying she'd never amount to much if she were overweight. She couldn't move past that set of thoughts. She couldn't know herself beyond her body. She believed she *was* her body, forgetting about her intelligence, charm, and kindness and her willingness to move mountains to help another.

The body is a wonderful vehicle integral to who you are, but it's not all of who you are, and Maxi wasn't getting that. She believed if she were thin, she'd be happy. If she were thin, she wouldn't be judged. If she were thin, she would be lovable. If she were thin, she'd be laughing and joking, and happy as could be, like her two friends.

So, after this lovely weekend, a barrage of texts poured into my phone from Maxi who'd recently returned home from her "dream vacation." She was back and miserable, reliving every moment of her trip, from her view. Maxine had dreamt of this trip for months on end, imagining how great getting away from the office and hanging out with two best friends from childhood would be—and having a few cheat days—because, well she deserved it.

But while in sunny California, she couldn't accept the fact that she was beyond her body. She believed she *was* her body. And here she was in this amazing state of sunshine, palm trees, and sandy beaches, wishing to be home working where she felt useful and productive, even if she didn't feel she had an opportunity for a higher position. But the truth of the matter is while she was at work, she dreamt of being anywhere but there.

A Trip to the Ocean

Maxi reminded me of a story I once heard in one of my college classes. The professor was speaking about this fellow who was at the office dreaming about spending time at the beach. The fellow closed his eyes, took a deep breath and imagined the sounds of the waves washing along the shoreline, the smell of sweet ocean air, and seagulls squawking to the beat of the day.

So pleasant was this guy's visual, to maintain it at the forefront of his mind, he kept a rather large conch shell he'd scooped up years before on a diving trip to remind him of the ocean. Many times throughout the day, he'd pick up his shell pressing it close against his ear to hear the sound of the sea.

Though, of course, he wasn't really listening to the ocean, but rather he heard the noise of the surrounding environment resonating within the cavity of the shell—but the sound took him there anyway. He'd daydream, imagining a frolic at the beach, carefree and free of the hustle bustle of work, smiling at the mere idea of such a getaway.

And then this very fellow finally set off for a well-planned journey to the ocean—a place that brought him pure joy, a place he imagined himself to be every day at work. So here he was, well on his way to having that wonderful experience he dreamt of so often at the office. Soon he was sprawled out on the beach after a long day of diving, with his entire set of beach necessities, wanting for nothing, yet all he could think about was what he was missing at the office.

This is exactly what Maxi was doing, *sort of*. She had been dreaming about this luxurious vacation in sunny California, away from work responsibilities, yet when she arrived there, she was miserable and thinking about work and what she might be missing. And now she was home, and guess what? She was miserable.

What was going on here? Maxi missed the memo: ***Every Day Is a Good Day!***

No matter where you go, or whom you're with, you're going to bring yourself along. If you're miserable here, you most likely will be miserable there. Maxi hated her body, her life, and who she was right here at home; hence, that's what she brought with her to sunny California. *Wherever you go—there you are.*

Are you making every day a good day? Or are you dreaming about that vacation while you're working? And then when you're on vacation, are you thinking about what you're missing at home?

Dial into a Greater Channel

Maxi, and most of us for that matter, needs to dial into a greater channel of who we really are. If we're hyper-focused on our bodies and not being physically what we think we should be, we may well be missing out on the moment. The physical reality might be blocking the spiritual reality.

The gift of life, and of being, can be blocked by this physical wish. The greater reality of who we are is well beyond the body—and for sure beyond the food.

Maxi remained in her negative view of her body, based on how she judged her body—and how she thinks others are judging her. And in this case, one of the girlfriends did make reference to the fact that Maxi had gained weight, and she did so right there at the restaurant while Maxi was indulging in a fried-food concoction she thought she deserved—because she was on vacation.

Her friend's comment reinforced Maxi's shame and judgment of herself, that she was no good, and didn't deserve to be happy, and that she'd amount to nothing *if she was fat.*

Maxi felt awful eating foods she knew weren't on her healthy eating plan, and then when her friend told her that she was worried about her, the further comment only made matters worse. Maxi plummeted into a deep, dark hole of despair. Maxi already did a fine job of shaming and blaming herself for her life not turning out the way that she'd dreamed, and now she had the notion hooked, packaged, and delivered that she was a failure—*just as her dad told her she would be.*

Maxi was comparing, judging, and shaming herself, and the girlfriend's observation only compromised any opportunity of making every day a good day.

So what was Maxi to do? That she'd gained weight was true, but this thought became her sole experience of the trip. She couldn't erase this line of thinking that she wasn't good enough, pretty enough, or thin enough—so as this fear gripped her, she ate more. Food served as a pacifier for her, at least for the moment, until the shame and blame and judging kicked in.

Maxi and I spent many sessions to clear out her faulty belief system as we worked on her being able to see her lovely qualities. She began to realize she didn't have to be thin to begin to love herself—and that she could allow herself to grow into the size she was meant to be—whatever that size would be.

With work and over time, Maxi began to heal that panicky space in her mind and understand that she wasn't her body, and that her friend wasn't trying to hurt her, but was actually concerned about her wellbeing due to the weight gain. Her judging, shaming, and blaming herself for picking up the weight wasn't going to bring Maxi into a happy, *every day is a good day* space. Instead, she had to feel the pain and move through it rather than eating it and keeping it down. On the trip, Maxi distracted herself from the pain by eating foods that simply weren't good for her, only making herself feel worse.

Bolstered by our sessions together, Maxi regrouped and began to work on self-loving through bringing in healthy real foods, exercising, and changing her negative thoughts to positive ones. She realized eating processed foods on her California trip had made her feel anxious and bloated, and ignited her pattern of judging, shaming, and blaming.

Maxi tended to blame and shame herself as she relived her childhood fears of not fitting in, or not being liked in this adult life while in the company of these very same girls in *their* now-adult life. Her feelings from back then had never healed, and seeing the friends and hanging out with them in the town where this blueprint had been set down reignited her fears.

Awareness

The only way for Maxi to emerge from this funk was to become conscious of what she was doing. She began to stop and ask herself why she felt so awful when she was around those childhood friends. And sparks of memory popped up regarding their childhood lives versus hers. Maxi's parents were divorced, and according to Maxi she'd lived on the poor side of town, whereas her two friends lived in lovely homes on the rich side of town, and their parents' relationships were intact. They had *real* families not fractured ones like Maxi's.

On this trip, Maxi had regressed back to being the little girl she was then, and not the powerful girl she had turned into. She wasn't accepting who she was these days and opening her heart to be compassionate with herself. She didn't know how to unpack what she was feeling. Now, she realized she was living her best life working in a field of meaning and making an income that allowed her to feel good about her accomplishments.

Maxi recognized that she had gained some weight and mentioned how that made her feel despair, self-hatred, and self-disgust, but this was prompted by the childhood message that she was poor and not as good as her wealthy friends. She wasn't tapping into the Divine nature of who she really was—a kind, loving, good person—beyond her body size.

Maxi began to realize, accept, and most important, believe she could go on a trip and have a lovely time regardless of her size, that she needed to embrace the now of where she was, not the tomorrow of who she wanted to be. ***Acting as if*** she might be able to free herself of where she'd been stuck for years and years was the beginning of her healing.

It wasn't Maxi's girlfriend who'd opened up the shame and blame and judging of Maxi, because she had been doing this long before her friend made the comment. And the comment wasn't made to be cruel but came from a loving place.

Okay, I hear you saying, Are you kidding? The friend wasn't nice making reference to Maxi's weight. Well, on the surface that may seem true, but the friend didn't offer her remark out of anger or cruelty, but rather out of love. Maxi has a family history of heart disease and diabetes—both parents passed away at young ages because they didn't practice self-love and take care of their health. They were living the way Maxi was living, but without awareness. Maxi is now aware and has opportunity for change, and her friend was trying to point this out.

As Maxi began the process of forgiving herself for not unconditionally loving herself, and for judging herself, she blossomed like a sunflower, tall and erect, reaching to the sky. She began to tap into her Divine self, which is beyond her body. She began to self-forgive for not loving and caring for herself. As Maxi began to self-forgive, she began to heal from the inside out.

You, too, can begin to heal from the inside out. You can begin the process of self-love, just as Maxi did. You can go on vacation and be totally fine with yourself exactly as you are, in the body where you currently reside. Your real issue isn't the shape of your body, its appearance; the real concern needs to be on your self-care and your self-love.

Take the first step, and your mind will mobilize all its forces to your aid. Once the battle is started, all that is within and without you will come to your assistance. Every day is a good day—if you want it to be. Even when times are tough, focus on the smallest things such as the breath still in you.

Personal Inventory Questions

1. Every day presents a new opportunity to make the day a good one, no matter what happened yesterday, last week, last year, or a lifetime ago. Every day is a good day no matter where you are: London, Italy, France, Tennessee, or at home on a long weekend. Do you believe this to be true?
2. *Take the first step, and your mind will mobilize all its forces to your aid.* Ah, but you might say, how can I take the first step when I'm so tired, when my mind is bogged down with the weight of life? All your transformation requires is that first try, and change will come rushing in. What first step do you need to take?
3. Perhaps you wish for tomorrow, or that vacation, or a long weekend, or you remember a better yesterday, or a wonderful time last year, or when you were younger. But is your wish really for tomorrow, or for better times right at this moment?
4. If you recall when Maxi texted to tell me she wasn't doing so great, she couldn't pinpoint why. She knew she felt really sad and anxious but claimed those emotions had come up for no apparent reason. Upon closer examination she saw she had plenty of reasons for feeling sad. Do you ever feel

anxious and sad for no apparent reason? If so, perhaps a closer look will unveil what is truly going on.

5. Remember how Maxi felt trapped in her job; with no room to move up, no love life, and nothing to look forward to, alongside memories of her father saying she'd never amount to much if she were overweight? These memories stirred and grew shame, blame, and judgment within her. Can you recall having such feelings, or know where they might have been ignited?
6. Maxi was comparing, judging, and shaming herself, and the girlfriend's comment only compromised any opportunity of making every day a good day. What comments were made to you that compromised your opportunity of making every day a good day?
7. Is it possible every day can be a good day even in a difficult time?
8. What about the fellow picking up the conch seashell from his desk, pressing it against his ear, which transported him to the ocean where he truly felt free and happy. And what about this very same fellow who was finally at the ocean wishing to be at work? Do you do this?
9. Maxi began to realize, accept, and most important, believe she could go on a trip and have a lovely time regardless of her size—that she needed to be present in the now of where she was, not the tomorrow of who she wanted to be. Can you accept and believe you can go on a trip and have a lovely time regardless of your size?
10. As Maxi began the process of forgiving herself for not unconditionally loving herself and for judging herself, she blossomed like a sunflower, tall and erect, reaching to the sky. She began to tap into her Divine self that is beyond her body. Can you tap into your Divine self beyond your body?

Chapter 19

Eat Your Way Through Europe

Travel isn't always pretty.
It isn't always comfortable.
Sometimes it hurts,
It even breaks your heart.
But that's okay.
The journey changes you—it should change you.
It leaves marks on your memory, on your consciousness,
on your heart, and on your body.
You take something with you…
hopefully, you leave something good behind.
~Anthony Bourdain

Can you imagine a full-blown confirmed food addict heading out to Europe not eating sugar, flour, or wheat? Yep, I'm gong into the unknown, and I want to take you with me step by step…food by food.

Separate, well-thought-out, and orchestrated: clothes, shoes, bags, makeup, books, and toiletries, all laid out on the bed, ready to be packed. For weeks on end, I sorted and resorted my clothes until I had the *perfect* selections for my fourteen-day adventure. Now, all I had to do was arrange my choices in my suitcase. Simple, yes, but I had a problem. Only one-quarter of the items fit—and I had one hour left to pack and head to the airport. I pushed, pulled, folded, and shoved, all while Southern Grace, my curious white Swiss shepherd puppy, pressed her wet, black nose against each article, until she grabbed a blouse, and ran like the wind.

Panic set in with me not knowing what to take and what to abandon—knowing I had to leave most items behind. All that planning for naught, placing me in a whirl of worry. Husband Joe to the rescue. He gently waved me away and packed the essentials, forgetting the rest. And so, off we went to the airport. My first flight to Europe—*and alone.* All my people were waiting across the pond…

Bon Voyage

I boarded Norwegian Air to London mid-July at ten p.m., giddy with awe, wondering what Mom's relatives' land would present in England, and Dad's in Italy. With London my first stop, thoughts of tea, hats, and English accents danced in my head, and to my delight I was greeted by flight attendants wearing sleek and stylish uniforms. The men wore blue-checkered blazers and waistcoats, along with crisply pressed white shirts and dark-blue ties, while the women were outfitted in elegantly designed dark-blue dresses; cardigans; white blouses; and adorable dark-blue, fedora-type hats propped straight atop their heads and decorated with deep-red ribbon around the base, complemented by scarves around their necks, draping down the front of the cardigan. And red gloves to polish the look.

I was in awe. The uniforms were so British.

I made my way to the very last seat on the entire plane. *Goodness,* I thought, *this can't be good.* The very last seat next to the toilet was where I'd be spending my next eight-plus hours.

And this spot proved to be delightful. No seats were taken on the last three rows, so I sprawled out with my books, laptop, and Italian lessons, along with the prepared foods I carried with for the flight, and I settled in for what was my most relaxing travel experience *ever.*

All the warnings as to how awful my experience traveling to Europe would be were countered by my joyous crossing. I sipped my hot tea, watched two movies—a rare opportunity for me with my hectic life—ate roasted chicken, asparagus with a garlic butter sauce, and a sweet potato. After, filling my belly, I slept a good portion of the way. Life is good.

I was stoked to see London, followed by parts of Italy. I longed to understand these areas and hoped to fill in the blanks of what made my parents who they were, coming from these parts. I had no idea what I was up for, but now in hindsight, the journey was amazing.

Traveling through Europe was a life-changer for me. I will never forget my experiences *forever marked in my memory, in my consciousness, and most definitely in my heart and on my body. I did take something with me—something good and perhaps something bad as well.*

I'd never been to Europe before, so I didn't know what to expect. I'd thought I would fall in love with London, as my mom's entire family were Londoners, and Italy, I imagined, would simply be a sidebar. But that's not what happened. Italy is forever engraved in my heart. My dad's family was there—and some still are—in the small town of Duvelle, outside of Vicenza.

The months preceding my trip were filled with the emotions of both excitement and fear. I'd never left my family for two weeks before, which included my new puppy, Southern Grace, who at that time was only five months old, and my eclectus parrot Oliver, along with my husband, and our oldest son.

I worried that they'd struggle without me. I was concerned how I'd find the foods I needed—as for the first time in traveling I wasn't able to carry most of it, or at least the essentials, until I arrived at my destination, which this time was foreign *for real.* And to top off my concerns, I'd saddled my husband with a project I set up with our handyman from the west coast of Florida. Eric would stay at our home the entire time and install new flooring.

I know, I know—that doesn't sound very fair. But the arrangement seemed perfect. Eric is amazing with parrots, so Oliver would be released from his cage for exercise, and my sweet puppy would have company every day as Eric was bringing his nine-year-old with him. A win-win, I thought—while I traipsed around Europe!

So I left with a quantity of guilt, but mostly, to be honest, worry about how I'd fit in my morning walk and eat healthy foods every four to five hours, a ritual I'd followed for the past twenty-plus years to quiet my eating disorder.

Normally, when I travel I bring muffins and other goodies to tide me over until I hit a store upon arrival. But now I was trekking to Europe, with no clue where I could shop, or even how I'd get to the stores, not to mention speak the language in Italia.

After I checked in at the airport, I said goodbye to Joe and went through security, then into the restricted lounge.

Prior to our boarding, I whipped out my journal and began to write:

July 16, 2016
~England/Italy Bound~

> *I'm off to Europe—with mixed feelings. I should be excited, but I'm stressed. We arrived early enough, but parking was an issue.*
> *My bag was 100 percent full. Joe had randomly pulled and packed a pile of clothes for me from among those items I'd so carefully gathered—so now I'm sure I won't have big choices.*
> *I'm here at the airport waiting. I'm wound up—huge headache, and I don't have my planned foods with me except for my airplane foods. I had no room in my bag. So, for real, I'm in the Hands of God. I'm going it the way Father Rookey always said—without a plan—just knowing that the right foods will be available. God works that way. Fr. Peter Mary Rookey, O.S.M. was a Servite friar in the Roman Catholic Church, widely believed to have had the charisma of healing, and he spent a good part of his priesthood in that ministry. He was born October 12, 1916 and passed on September 10, 2014, one day after my birthday. I was blessed to know him and wrote about him extensively in my first book: Release Your Obsession with Food: Heal from the Inside Out.*
> *Once on the plane I can let go…*
> *My goal is to chronicle daily my food and experience while in Europe.*

So here I soon was, this late Wednesday night at 10 p.m. on my flight to London, leaving all those worries behind, with only brief moments of wondering how everything was turning out back home. Goodbye palm trees, goodbye ocean, goodbye Florida.

Once escorted all the way to the very back of the plane, I found my seat equipped with a screen to watch a movie, and plug-ins to use my iPad, computer, and iPhone. I was set.

A Good Book Goes a Long Way

Settled in my seat, I whipped out *Memoirs of a Solo Traveler: My Love Affair with Italy,* written by Margie Miklas, which remained my constant touchstone throughout my trip, offering morsels of information, experiences, and comedic interactions with the beautiful Italian community.

Some of my experiences mirrored Margie's, such as meeting my relatives, looking for family landmarks, plus discovering the antiquated ways of the post office, that businesses closed between one and three p.m., not to mention trying to speak Italian in different dialects, all of which enhanced my enjoyment and didn't disappoint. The author paints her respect and understanding of the Italian people and culture, which flavored my own expectations and personal experience.

Unlike Margie Miklas, for me, the trip started in London in the quaint town of Esher, where I was to stay with my niece Jacqueline; her husband, Trevor, and three children, at their home; along with my sister Mickey and her husband, Emil, who are visiting as well from Illinois. The plan was to stay in London Wednesday until Saturday, then fly to Italy for one week, and then back to London for a few days, and then back to Florida for me, and Illinois a week later for my sister Mickey and husband.

In London at Gatwick Airport, I made my way to customs but had no idea where I was going. Wide-eyed, looking like an American tourist, when they asked for an address, I was totally stumped. I relied on the fact that Jacqueline, my niece, was picking me up, and had never thought beyond that.

A very stern customs agent repeated, "Where are you going?" I repeated I had no idea, that my niece was picking me up, and that this was my first time in Europe. I received stares up and down. My face flushed with sweat beading on my forehead, upper lip, and chin, and dripping down my back—my sheer panic turned to fear. I felt I was in trouble.

But then I excused myself from the line—amid stares and grunts from the annoyed travelers behind me, and stepped aside, frantically fumbling for my phone. Grateful for Facebook, I tracked Jacqueline through messenger, where she gave me her address. I was free to go.

A Taste of London

London was amazing. The air was fresh, cool, and clean, and the accent was icing on the cake. The greenery, blooming flowers, and exquisite skyline ever-etched themselves in my mind. I felt good. Esher is a town in Surrey, England, to the east of the River Mole. An outlying suburb of London, with Esher Commons at its southern end, the town marks one limit of the built-up Greater London area. One of the attractions is the mainline station at Esher, which provides fast, regular service to London Waterloo, while both freeways, the M25 and A3, are a short drive away.

I traveled with four adults and three young children, eight of us in total. I walked around bug-eyed in amazement, and in awe of how people lived across the pond throughout our trip, except in London, a girl's outing.

Everything was surreal—but the food was the same. I saw fast foods on just about every corner in London. The city reminded me of Chicago, and I heard others say New York. It had that same "city" feel.

Finding food that fit my needs was easy everywhere we traveled in London. Salads were plentiful as were fruits, starchy unprocessed carbs, fats, and dairy. The only food that seemed quite pricey were the proteins. This was the first time in a long time I had the feeling that I wouldn't have enough to eat. And at times, once in Italy, I wasn't able to eat an ample amount when protein was factored in—and often fruit was lacking too, with the exception of those I carried with me, and those sold on the streets from carts.

In London, we ran into castles everywhere. Windsor Castle, in the town of Windsor—the queen's preferred residence in London—as we learned, is the largest and oldest occupied castle in the world, the original castle having been built in the eleventh century. Somewhere along the way, we witnessed a changing-of-the-guard ceremony near Buckingham Palace, the place most people think of when they think of the British Royal Family. This is the official Royal Residence of the monarch, and has been since Queen Victoria came to the throne and moved there from Kensington Palace.

At Buckingham Palace, the queen creates knights, holds state banquets, receives ambassadors, and performs all sorts of other royal duties. Some of them are televised, including grand meetings between the many international dignitaries with The Queen herself.

My internal clock had me at my "normal" times, even though a time difference was at play. Each morning, I was up by six-fifteen a.m. just as I would be at home, and I went off to sleep around midnight. I think keeping my days and meals at the same intervals contributed to the ease of working my food in each day. I also attribute my comfort to the light and dark controlling my waking hour and sleep. When the light streamed through the window, I was up and out, propped at the table, sipping tea, writing in a quiet space while everyone else slept.

Once the group was up and about—free of jet lag—on the second day, my sister, twelve-year-old great niece, Jacqueline my niece, and I made our way to London for the day on Friday—as Thursday had been a recuperation-from-jet-lag, get-acclimated kinda day. We were then off to the train: there known as the *tube*. Even though the system is called the tube, meaning the underground, about half of the system is above ground. The "Tube" is a slang name for the London underground, because the tunnels for some of the lines are round tubes running through the ground. I can still hear, "Mind the gap!" every time we exited—a warning to watch the space between the train itself and the platform.

In London, we walked and walked, and walked some more. One of my concerns on this trip (as noted in my diary) was that I wouldn't fit in my morning exercise. Well, that was never, ***ever*** an issue the entire trip. On and on we walked, to the point that my toes were really sore, cramping, and blistered. Yes, I bought a really swanky pair of new sneakers to wear about *without breaking them in.*

After gallivanting around London with our tour guide, Steven, a good looking fortyish guy with golden hair, sporting a trimmed mustache and beard, and dressed in a light olive-green, plaid suit jacket; crisp white shirt; red-and-black tie matching the dark lapel to his jacket; and black pants, and carrying a black umbrella having a hook handle, and that he often held in the air to keep his posse together. He was comical and knowledgeable all rolled into one.

I was soon to learn that London, the capital of England and of the United Kingdom, is a twenty-first-century city with history stretching back to Roman times. As we marched along at the city center, we feasted upon: the Houses of Parliament, the iconic "Big Ben" clock tower, and Westminster Abbey—the site of British monarch coronations.

We stood gazing out across the Thames River, where we could see the London Eye, which we didn't have time for—but I was told this observation wheel provides panoramic views of the South Bank cultural complex and the entire city.

Of course, we couldn't walk around London without poking into castles such as Buckingham Palace, which was a sight to behold. The charming red phone booths scattered about in London-Westminster still stand, reminding me of how far we've come with technology, each of us carrying our own device.

We passed the Churchill War Rooms, and shortly after, the horse guard parade, and then St. James Park, loaded with exquisite greenery and flowers of every color imaginable. Then we strolled through The Mall, soaking up more trees and foliage as the ceremonial marching band went by in their full red jackets, black pants, and black hat attire, with what looked to me like animal fur on top. I wondered how they could see with their hats so low. The royal band with its trumpets blaring, symbols clanging, and drums drumming was a sight to see.

The horse guards are guarded by both mounted and foot troopers from the Household Calvary. My understanding was that two mounted troopers were on post daily between ten a.m. and four p.m. during the summer months. These troopers are relieved every hour. We caught the new guard riding in at Buckingham Palace and Constitution Hill—a perfect spot for photos, thanks to Steven, our tour guide.

We seemed to run into the magnificent guard almost as if we were following the parade all the way to Whitehall, and seeing the entire ceremony. Whitehall is in Central London, the main entrance to which is partway between Downing Street and Trafalgar Square. The smell of horses, greenery, and other perfumes all blended into a heavenly scent.

Cars whizzed by on the "wrong" side of the road, something that made me dizzy to the point I had to close my eyes as a passenger. The side they drove on just didn't seem right. Did I mention we were with my great niece, at the time twelve years old, leading us through the city, totally dependent on her as Jacqueline left us early in the morning to work?

Vanessa, well beyond her years, with the help of her smartphone navigated our way to a lovely café, where we finally ate. I was now starving, though we had eaten a filling breakfast only hours before.

At the lovely café in the Mayfair area of Westminster, I ate salad filled with tomatoes, a spring mix of baby greens, spinach, and kale, along with chunks of chicken, red bell peppers, tomatoes, and with a lovely red vinegar and olive oil dressing on top.

Afterward, we enjoyed cups of decaffeinated cappuccino. As in the States, I paid with my cash and tipped with a handful of pretty, colorful coins of different amounts, not realizing I was paying triple the amount of what I needed to, thinking the coins were just loose change, like here in the US.

Every day, thus far, all my foods had been clean, meaning whole, fresh, real, and on task. My nephew Trevor, an excellent cook, grilled steaks to perfection with oven-roasted garlic, olive oil potatoes, and roasted asparagus one night, and grilled breasts of chicken to equal perfection with baked potatoes, roasted-garlic broccoli, peppers, and mushrooms on another night. Though the meals were excellent, the best part was bonding while sharing conversation and laughter, and creating memories of a lifetime.

Breakfasts were eggs made into a quiche filled with vegetables, cheese, tomatoes, and onions, along with red raspberries, bananas, and oatmeal, accompanied by hot tea laced with almond milk.

I started off right, and my sticking to my foods kept going day after day, proving you *can* eat clean, no matter where you are, or what's going on—and not feel deprived. We have a choice.

Italia Here We Come

One of the most frustrating things in traveling is packing way too much. I know you're thinking, but you said your husband took away three-quarters of your clothes. Yes he did. But my suitcase was still too full!! And when you're packing and unpacking your things, which we did as we traveled about, doing that with so much in a bag can be quite difficult. And to buy anything to bring back was a no-no because I had no room—*or money*…another story to come.

Arranging my possessions before heading off to Italy from England, I once again had no room in my suitcase for anything extra. Note to self: This seems to be a common thread in my life. Stuff…too much stuff. Less is more…

On Saturday, only days after my arrival in England, we made our way to Venice, landing at the Marco Polo Airport. The airport is located on the mainland four-point-three nautical miles north of the city in Tessera, a small village near Venice, close to Mestre.

The terminal is not only architecturally stunning, but it's also equipped with a state-of-the-art security system. Nearly tripping over my feet and luggage, I captured dramatic pictures of the airport floor—the art was exquisite. This was only a small taste of things to come as the days in Italy unfolded.

The three kids, my sister's grandchildren, pulled luggage through the airport like troopers, as they were accustomed to traveling throughout Europe, while Mickey and I—and Emil too—were innocents, excited to soak it all in. The instant I exited the plane, I felt the shift—different country—different culture. Once again, I had to manage my way through customs, but this time I was with experienced travelers and felt more at ease.

Our first stop was to secure our rented extra-long vehicle, big enough to accommodate our little posse for our travels throughout Northern Italy, as we had many stops planned. *Well, not so easy*. We waited, and waited, *and waited*—welcome to Italy where "no rush" appeared to be the constant message—as *The Memoir of a Solo Traveler* mentions throughout.

The kids were hot since the temperature was nearing ninety degrees, and hungry, and so was I. Did I mention I become super crabby when I don't eat for hours on end? Hence, my fear of not having my foods with me comes to mind…

In Italy, we stayed in a cottage three-hundred-forty feet above sea level on a mountainside, where the air was thin, leaving challenges for me so far as breathing was concerned—but the beauty far surpassed any distress I suffered.

Winding our way up and down the mountain was trying, to say the least. I feared our over-large vehicle would fall off the cliff. The only comfort I had was in knowing Trevor was driving on the right side of the road and positioned "per normal" in the car—less dizzying for me than driving on the opposite side of the road in England.

But fear remained with me on our ups and downs every time we returned to our lovely cottage. The mountain roads had no barriers on the side and no dividing line for oncoming traffic.

Hiking and *walking and walking and walking* filled up the majority of our time. But I loved our little country bungalow up in the mountains, totally secluded, with only Italian-speaking people around.

Upon arrival, we made our way to a market in the village. Nobody spoke a word of English, while we struggled with our phone translations, receiving many sighs and much eye-rolling from the Italians. We were exhausted and starving, and realized we needed our staples to last us through the first day until we could make our way to the *real* grocery store—which looked like a mall to me.

The *real* store, *Centro Commerciale Di Abano,* was housed with other mini-stores inside the main structure. I felt as though I was in a mall with a grocery store positioned in such a way you could see the activities happening in the other stores, such as Le Flamboyant, Alidiro, Non Solo Spot (sneakers), an eyeglass shop, a hair salon, and a jewelry store, to name a few.

The key to traveling—anywhere in the world—is to prepare in advance, to stop at a store or market to obtain food and drink supplies to carry you through your journey without your having to resort to fast foods or foods that won't promote health, but will rather lead you down the path of guilt, shame, and self-judging, not to mention cheat days.

Once you've eaten nutritious foods, you'll begin to feel confident that having the most amazing travel experience is possible and probable, placing the focus on the now and soaking in the culture, rather than the cheat foods that can take over and make the trip a nightmare.

I know, I can hear you saying, "But the food in the culture IS the experience." Yes, this is true. But the food doesn't have to be sugar, flour, and wheat. It can be fruits, vegetables, lean proteins, high-quality fats, non-processed starchy carbs, and dairy. Think about what that can mean. Pull those foods together for an amazing feast such as fruits and yogurt, or steak with roasted potato and a salad topped with tomatoes and fresh mozzarella.

Italians eat close to the Mediterranean style with loads of vegetables, olive oil, fruits, and fish. Cappuccinos can be found on almost every corner for a "pick-me-up." In most of the "touristy" spots, finding bottled water and fresh fruits was easy. I also carried with me a trail mix of nuts, organic crackers made of sprouts, and raisins for emergencies if I was becoming hungry. And for long car rides, I carried a cooler with fruits, boiled eggs, and raw veggies, should I need a fix.

Terre Bianche

At the cottage, Terre Bianche, known as "*the cottage in the park*," where we spent seven glorious days in Teolo, Italy, we were greeted by Angela, an eloquent, red-headed Italian—owner of the Airbnb, who seemed to be always dressed elegantly, with jewelry and hair intact, even while she was bent over picking the vegetation on her land.

Up on the mountain, we roamed the terrain, finding fresh olives, apples, raspberries, and grapes, and tiny pears that provided an amazing snack. We ate out on the terrace every evening at a long table with a breathtaking view of mountains around us. Cooking facilities were available to us, making evening meals easy, together with easy preparations to load up on good foods for our next day's travels. During our stay at the villa, we had a stove, grill, and refrigerator, along with a large walk-in pantry.

Our first attempt at dining at a restaurant in the little town of Teolo was hilarious. Nobody understood English, and we didn't understand Italian. I had studied for a few months, thinking I was good to go. Not. My poor language skills were embarrassing, to say the least, but we managed to be fed.

After fumbling through the ordering process I finally ordered a succulent steak, fresh Brussels sprouts in a buttery sauce, roasted potatoes, and sparkling water—*acqua frizzante*—which they brought to the table in large bottles. I preferred the fizzy one as it was refreshing and filling.

After waiting for what felt like an eternity, our incredible meals arrived—but mine was missing the roasted potatoes. Try as I might to catch the waiter's attention, he ignored me. I guess he was annoyed. To this day, my brother-in-law shares the story—especially the part of my not getting my potatoes after what seemed like an hour's process of trying to order my food.

I woke each day in Italy long before the others, enjoying my quiet out on the terrace, writing, meditating, praying, and journaling, listening to the locusts make a swishing musical melody, at times super loud—while the church bells chimed on schedule, on the hour every hour.

Most mornings I had eggs, blueberries, and oatmeal. Preparation was simple, and the food worked into healthy eating. That early in the day, I sat out at a picnic table overlooking the mountains, writing and sipping on my coffee that I'd made using a little percolator that I heated on the stove, taking more than THIRTY minutes to brew. I wanted to feel the realness without the microwave comforts…all while the others slept.

Out for an Outing

In Arqua Petrarca, a small town in northeastern Italy, in the Veneto region, the province of Padua, I felt that time stood still. In this quaint town, the center of the Euganean Hills, the locals said that more than any other village around, this town maintained the charm of the medieval. I picked a loose rock off a wall to transport home…one of the oldest rocks used to build here, they claimed.

For every outing, I packed my needed foods and water—*just in case*—as my sister reminded me. She couldn't bear my troubled moods when I didn't eat—as she continually reminded me. And little Colty was mesmerized and obsessed by my things, snatching my headband, and prancing around like a bunny, wearing it as he grinned from ear to ear. He also liked looking in my food bag and taking bites of my snacks and swigs of my water—leaving behind a little backwash.

Venice Here We Come

Venice (*Venezia*) is a city in northeastern Italy and the capital of the Veneto region. It's situated on a group of one-hundred-eighteen small islands that are separated by canals and linked by over four-hundred bridges. We witnessed the beauty of this locale firsthand, visiting the collage of Venice including the Piazza San Marco, the Grand Canal, and the interior of the opera house La Fenice, as well as taking in a view of the island of San Giorgio Maggiore. All spectacular.

Our time in Venice was amazing, especially when we rode in the gondolas, though they weren't as imagined, with no music playing and no romance. The water was a murky green and the paddler didn't seem to enjoy moving us about as he maneuvered under the Rialto Bridge through Venice's main water thoroughfare lined with great renaissance palaces and returning around the back streets of Venice.

We walked the streets of Venice and then to St. Mark's Square, la Piazza, where we ate a lovely salad filled with dark greens, shavings of fresh Parmesan cheese, tomatoes, and chicken. After our bellies were full, we checked out Rio di San Salvador, lined with beautiful churches, particularly the Chiesa di San Salvatore (of the Holy Savior), a church along the Merceria, the main shopping street of Venice.

Parts of Venice were a bit eerie…walls too close, making us feel claustrophobic. And seeing clothes hanging on lines to dry seemed quite barbaric. We learned that the city continues sinking—at a slow rate of one to two millimeters per year, with a state of alert in place.

We walked in and out of many churches and cathedrals, like the Basilica Dei Frari, St. Mark's Basilica (Basilica of San Marco), and the Chiesa di San Nicolò da Tolentino on the Rio del Tolentini. Passing smaller canals and passageways not visible from the city's narrow streets, we made our way back to the car. Along the route, we were impressed by so many frescoes—paintings, most of a holy moment, applied directly onto dry plaster imbedded on the wall, a refreshing sight, and not something you'd see on every street corner in the US.

The Family

The highlight of my trip in Northern Italy was in Dueville, meeting our relatives. We drove around and around, not knowing where we were going, to the point I began to feel my stomach gurgle, and fear gripped me because I had to use the bathroom soon. If you've ever been to Italy, you know the bathroom not only costs euros in some places, but often you have to squat as if you were in peasant times, *and the bathrooms are coed.*

Yes, you read right—both squat and coed. Squat because often the toilet was just a hole in the floor, and here I was with a serious stomach upset, and the facility was open to both male and female. The experience was not a pleasant one.

But the great part was that we finally found where we needed to be and waited in a quaint park for my cousin Annamaria to arrive. We heard out in the distance someone with a thick Italian accent yelling out, "Americanos, hello, hello, Americanos!" It was my cousin, who doesn't speak a lick of English and must have practiced those words for days, if not months.

Together we shared a pleasant meal with my dad's first cousin, Nico (Domenico); his wife, Elda; and Annamaria's parents and three sisters: Roberta, Anna, and Agatha—all distant cousins.

Again, the foods I needed were there…a delightful never-ending salad of tomatoes, carrots, cabbage, and greens; sizzling steak; fresh fruit; and my favorite, a bottle of Levico, Naturale, a fizzy water that I came to adore. Watching my dad's cousin interacting with Mikalina (my sister Mickey) was surreal, and we laughed and cried about the interaction for days on end afterward, because they talked, laughed, and squealed—yet neither spoke the other's language.

And then we went to Caldogno, a town and commune (the commune is an administrative division) near Vicenza, Italy, where my grandfather Nono lived until he moved to America with my grandmother, Nona Anna. In honor of the blessed mother, he built a monument out of marble, which I called a shrine. Four marble pillars surrounded steps leading up to a life-size Blessed Mary placed inside on a pedestal. Mary was dressed in white with a blue cape, hands folded to her chest in prayer. Bountiful flowers surrounded the shrine along with a meticulous mowed lawn. It's a place of worship to this day.

And then there is a Monte Ortigara, in the Province of Vicenza, where the Battle of Mount Ortigara was fought from June tenth through June twenty-fifth in 1917 between the Italian and Austro-Hungarian armies for possession of Mount Ortigara in the Asiago Plateau. I'd hoped to visit as we share the same name, and my father spoke of it often, but time would not permit.

Another highlight was at *La Ceramica VBC,* where we bought and shipped home some beautiful ceramics. That same day, we made our way to Bassano del Grappa, where we had an amazing lunch of mozzarella cheese, onions, corn, tomatoes, and greens topped with tuna. Afterward we visited Fiume Brenta (Bassano Del Grappa) in Veneto where the Brenta Riviera is the villa-lined land on either side of a waterway linking Venice to Padova.

Romeo and Juliet

One day we traveled to Verona, Centro Storico, the home of Romeo and Giuletta, some say. The balcony is still intact, with Juliet wannabes—old and young alike—climbing up for a photo. That evening we consumed another meal just as exquisite as our lunch, with whole green beans, chunks of mozzarella, tomatoes, black olives, and boiled eggs topped with tuna. I was happy, as was young Colty when he stood by the makeshift coliseum alongside soldier actors he could interact with.

And from there, we stopped at Lago Garda, where we took a boat ride, and Colty almost fell overboard climbing up on the rail out of curiosity, which caused quite an upset with the family clan. Of course, only an hour before boarding the boat, the kids each ordered a single serving of gelato, but the server was so taken by Colton he triple served him—which led to one wired little boy on a fast moving boat…

By the end of the next day, I began to feel quite concerned about my breathing. I felt as though my airways weren't quite open. I was coughing and seemed to have built up phlegm. I began to realize mountain life—high elevation—isn't good for me. I'd had untreated asthma as a kid and felt catapulted back to that time when I could barely breathe with my wheezing and coughing.

In spite of my not feeling well, we did make our way to see the church of St. Anthony in Paduva, which I talk about extensively in my second book, *Release Your Obsession with Diet Chatter: Heal from the Inside Out,* as my grandfather, Nono, had attended this church in Italy as well as St. Anthony in Chicago, a smaller version of the one in Italy, but patterned after it. I felt as if I were going back in time. Because I hadn't been to the one in Chicago since I was a little girl, this looked the same to me…big and miraculous. But a year later, I visited the one in Chicago again and realized from my adult view that the church was quite small.

Our last day in Teolo at the cottage, we hiked down the mountain and back up. I found this to be the hardest workout of the entire trip. At the top was a midway landing with an oversized rosary and a bench. I said out loud, "Who'd want to sit here?" Well, after completing the climb down and then back up, guess who was sitting on that bench eating wild berries. Yep, I sat where the monks of long ago sat, resting my aching legs.

Off to Roma

Leaving the quaint countryside, we hopped a train to Roma, the capital of Italy filled of hustle and bustle with a city feel. Two young travelers with skateboards popped in on the second stop, explaining to us that they were skating through Italy. The terrain was exquisite, and we passed beautiful farms and rolling hills. Only a few weeks later, this very landscape experienced an earthquake.

At this point of our trip, I became really homesick, missing my husband, sons Ben and Kris, daughter-in-law Zoe, and fur/feather kids too.

My sister Mickey looked out for me the entire time, always concerned about whether I had enough food to eat—as she surely knew the snarly me comes out when I'm not fed—so she avoided that at all cost.

I was totally exhausted, never having walked so much. My clothes were beginning to hang on me as I was dropping weight, though such was unintended.

In Rome, we stayed in an Airbnb in a high-rise. The renters had carved a hotel-style suite into a building filled with condos and old—very old—elevators with the chain and see-through bars. Mickey refused to get in and climbed what seemed like hundreds of steps to avoid this contraption.

We each had our own rooms, and breakfast was served to our rooms every morning. I fed on eggs, yogurt, and oatmeal. We suffered a shortage of fruit, but I was ready. The little pears I'd picked up in Teolo made staying on course easy.

The Vatican

Words cannot describe the awe I felt seeing the Papal Basilica of St. Peter in the Vatican—an Italian renaissance church in Vatican City—the papal enclave within the city of Rome. St. Peter's is the most renowned work of renaissance architecture and the largest church in the world. Regarded as one of the holiest Catholic shrines, St. Peter's is the burial site of Saint Peter—the first apostle among Jesus's apostles—and also the first bishop (pope) of Rome.

Another highlight of Rome was the Sistine Chapel, and words cannot do the experience justice. It is a chapel in the Apostolic Palace, the official residence of the pope in Vatican City. The fame of the Sistine Chapel lies mainly in the frescos that decorate the interior, most particularly the Sistine Chapel ceiling and The Last Judgment by Michelangelo covering the altar wall.

Another highlight, in addition to St. Peter's Cathedral, the Sistine Chapel, and the Coliseum was Ristorante Deoardo II, a place where the rich and famous are known to dine among the brightest, deepest pink decor. We were treated like royalty. The owner seemed to play all parts: cook, bartender, server, and entertainment, speaking in Italian mixed with English, almost as if he were reciting in a play.

The owner also took to Colty, as most do, giving him loads of attention, including a lovely fresh orange, and though a simple gesture, the acknowledgement was a delight for the boy. Again, we ate lovely salads and had a large bottle of Acqua Nepi—fizze (fizzy) water. My meal further consisted of pork chops cooked to perfection with cooked zucchini and eggplant baked in olive oil on a bed of dark greens. The kids seemed addicted to the Margarita pizzas throughout our entire stay. We were all happy!

We concluded our trip in Rome at the Trevi Fountain…tossing our coins backward, for certain to return once again. Jacqueline, Vanessa, and I ended our Rome stay, dining our last evening at the Sul Tett Tratteria while the others stayed in. The restaurant was all the way up on the building's rooftop terrace with a breathtaking panoramic view of the Vatican all in lights—a perfect way to say goodbye. We were told this was one of actor Dustin Hoffman's hangouts.

Arrivederci Italia…

A Last Peek in London

We returned to London, leaving Italy behind, and soon I'd return home. On our last day, we made our way to Windsor Castle for a complete tour before winding down. I then prepared for my trip back to the States.

Travel isn't always pretty and it isn't always comfortable, but it will change you. My plan when I'd first arrived in London was to exchange my money. Somehow, we never did. I'd brought with me an insane amount of money, an amount too embarrassing to reveal or to be walking around with. So I'd left most of it in a hiding spot in London at my niece's home. I was then just about penniless and felt like a kid asking my niece Jacqueline for an allowance, until I realized the power of a credit card.

Needless to say, I didn't spend much during the remainder of our trip. I returned home thirteen pounds lighter from all the walking and with a pocketful of money, as well as a sore toe. But my breathing was restored, and I have memories to cherish for a lifetime without needing a cheat day(s) to stand in my way of embracing the now.

Stay tuned for Chapter 20—final thoughts.

Personal Inventory Questions

1. Can you imagine a full-blown confirmed food addict heading out to Europe and not eating sugar, flour, or wheat? As I traveled through these unknown parts, I

wanted to take you with me step by step…food by food. What memories did my journey stir within you of your personal trips?

2. Travel isn't always pretty, and it isn't always comfortable, but it will change you. How have your travels changed you?
3. I boarded Norwegian Air to London mid-July at ten p.m., giddy with awe, wondering what Mom's relatives' land would present in England, and Dad's in Italy. Have you traveled back to your parents' parts? What was that like for you?
4. Getting food that fit my needs was easy everywhere we traveled. Salads were plentiful as were fruits, starchy unprocessed carbs, fats, and dairy. The only food I found quite pricey was the proteins. Do you feel assured you can find the foods you need to maintain your healthy eating while you travel?
5. Settled in my airplane seat, I whipped out *Memoirs of a Solo Traveler: My Love Affair with Italy,* written by Margie Miklas, which remained my constant companion, throughout my trip. What book do you recall as helping you navigate through foreign areas?
6. Up on the mountain in Teolo we roamed the terrain, finding fresh olives, apples, raspberries, grapes, and little pears that were amazing to eat. Have you ever happily come upon natural foods provided by the earth to sustain some of your food needs while away from home?
7. We walked the back streets of Venice San Marco and then walked to St. Mark's Square. There, we dined on a delicious salad filled with lovely dark greens, shavings of Parmesan cheese, tomatoes, and chicken. What clean foods mark your memory from your last big trip?
8. Sometimes with a group of eight, both adults and children, the matter of having enough space can be challenging. We

took the initiative of taking our space, as needed. Are you able to nurture yourself in a quiet space when you need to?

9. My family reunion with cousins who barely spoke English was bonding, nonetheless. Do you have memories of meeting long-lost relatives you never before met in person? What did that meeting tell you about yourself?
10. Praying at the shrine with the Madonna holding her child that my grandpa built and was so proud of was one of the most moving moments in my life. What moment marks your highlight in regard to traveling?

Chapter 20

Final Thoughts

Visualize this thing that you want.
See it, feel it, believe in it.
Make your mental blueprint, and begin to build.
~Robert Collier

Believe it, and you will see it in actuality. Robert Collier, one of the greatest influencers in my life, taught me through his book *Riches Within Your Reach!* to see it, feel it, believe in it—and to make my mental blueprint—and then begin to build. I knew at a very young age I wanted to write but I didn't know how my ambition would come to fruition. In my youth, I had an old-fashioned typewriter, and I'd start over and over with: *Once upon a time…*

But once upon a time didn't arrive until I was ready for it. And I was ready when I began to understand I had to visualize this thing that I wanted and plant the seeds and wait. And wait I did.

A Walkathon Surprise

I recall walking for the March of Dimes many, many years ago when my young son was barely three years old. I pushed him in a lightweight stroller, compact to carry with me wherever I went as I weaved in and out of the crowds that very hot spring day.

Sweat was drenching me from every pore of my body but I barely noticed, as I was intrigued by my unplanned-for walking partner. I marched alongside a woman whose name I don't even recollect. She was a Christian writer for the *Miami Herald*, who happened to fall into step with me. We talked the entire way. I told her of my dream to write but that I didn't know where to begin.

This wise woman, in her thirties as I was at the time, explained I needed to write about something I felt passion for, in order to fuel my words. I, at the time, was a single mom, broke, and without a job, with the exception of lecturing for Weight Watchers of Greater Miami. I had a college degree in political science that wasn't going to do much for me as I had given up the idea of continuing toward a career as a graduate-level paralegal, and had also quit law school after one summer session. The law was not my calling.

What was I to do? I really did briefly entertain the idea of being a pest exterminator. Okay, the idea went through my mind for a brief thirty seconds, but I was broke and desperate to make ends meet. And God knows we have plenty of creepy crawlers in South Florida.

So, there I was, briskly walking side by side with this inspirational writer who told me how to make my dream come true. Only weeks after our walkathon I applied to Barry University to study in a field the most important to me: social work with an emphasis on mental health at the Master's level. One of the top persons at Weight Watchers suggested I apply for a scholarship, which I'd never thought of on my own.

See It, Feel It, and Believe in It

Sister McLoughlin, now deceased, firmly rejected my request for financial aid, saying all the scholarships had been given out—that this wasn't the time of year to apply. For some reason, I felt a nudge within me to write her a personal note outlining the reasons I should receive a scholarship, even though they had no scholarships left to give.

A *Source* greater than I wrote that letter. I'm convinced of that. I felt as if my hand moved across the pages powered by a force beyond that used in mere writing, leaving on the paper the most eloquent words one could produce from the heart.

I received a full scholarship the first year and two partials the remaining time I went to school there. I'm sure this was no coincidence. This was the movement of the Universe—a touch of an angel. I saw it and I believed it and it came—*when the time was right.*

At Barry, I wrote, researched, and studied everything about eating disorders and mental health while I worked for Weight Watchers of Greater Miami. I loved my job, my university, and my little boy who I was raising single handedly at the start of my education quest. I learned more about myself as I delved into a subject close to my heart, recognizing I did, in fact, have an eating disorder and that I needed to work on resolving my issue.

At some point during this period, I joined a twelve-step group and began to work on my food addiction. Post graduation, I started my therapy practice, and after a year, I reluctantly let go of my (thirteen-year by then) stint with Weight Watchers. Leaving a company that had helped me to initially lose one hundred pounds of weight was scary, but I kept bingeing, so I knew I needed more than this avenue to *fix* my problem. I also knew many people out *there* were just like me and needed a helping hand beyond being given a diet plan.

After graduating and practicing for a good ten years, I went on to obtain a doctoral degree and later earned a doctorate in addiction psychology, with the emphasis on food addiction. And then, finally, my writing career began to bloom, first with my dissertation, which just about wrote itself. The lovely walking partner, on that very hot fall day, had pushed me in the direction I needed to go with her wise words—and I never saw her again. But I never forgot her—another angel in my life.

My dissertation words were from the heart—from the soul—and from the qualitative research I delved into with every morsel of my being. I knew then I had to transform that academic piece into something simpler and more user-friendly after graduation—hence, ***Release Your Obsession with Food: Heal from the Inside Out*** was birthed. But after launching that book—the very last day I was with my beloved dad before he transitioned—I knew that was only the start of my writing career.

One year later, ***Release Your Obsession with Diet Chatter: Heal from the Inside Out*** launched. And now, you're holding in your hands, ***Release Your Obsession with Cheat DAZE: Heal from the Inside Out***... book three. But that's not the end—it's only the beginning. My next project, ***Release Your Obsession with Ageing: Heal from the Inside Out*** is in the works to be launched in 2020—a nice clean year for a new beginning.

Visualize This Thing That You Want

So imagine it's your birthday, Christmas, Chanukah, or a long holiday weekend, or that you're somewhere in Italy, wandering the streets with all kinds of tantalizing aromas whirling around in the air, but you're okay—no more cheat-day food frenzy, "gotta have it" kind of mania knocking at your mental door. No more, "If I just lost x-number of pounds..."

What would you feel like waking up day after day, anyplace at any time in your life, and eating in a "normal" way, with no head talk and no guilt and no cravings—being perfectly aligned with a healthy way of eating no matter where you are, who you're with, or what's going on in your life. And imagine further that you feel no gripping "willpower" or guilt, or jonsing, or any of those other old, familiar feelings when that *feeling* comes on, and you know you're going to cave.

You have to visualize this thing you want, like writing in my case, long before I mastered my cheat-day attitude. I believed in the core of my being that when I was ready, this dream would be my reality—but that I had to wait. I had to release my obsessions to open myself to my wants without a gripping, negative hold.

A very kind and gentle patient was surprised I'd never read the classic novel *Siddhartha*, by Hermann Hesse, a short story of self-discovery—a young Brahmin's quest for the ultimate reality. Shortly after, my patient gifted me said book, a powerful little volume that left me pondering about life and obsessions—a subject I write about at length. I'd like to share with you one short paragraph:

Siddhartha

"When someone seeks," Siddhartha said, "it is all too easy for his eyes to see nothing but the thing he seeks, so that he is unable to find anything because he is always thinking exclusively about what he seeks, because he has a goal, because he is obsessed by that goal. Seeking means having a goal. But finding means being free, remaining accessible, having no goal. You, venerable one, are perhaps really one who seeks, because pressing after your goal, you fail to see many a thing that is right before your eyes."

Visualizing the thing you want—to see it, feel it, believe in it, and to make your mental blueprint and build is *not* the same as being obsessed by that goal. Remember finding means being free. To obsess over a cheat day—being "allowed" to eat a highly processed food—is not freedom, but rather makes it all too easy for your eyes to see nothing but this thing you seek.

Living your life obsessing over the one day you can eat whatever you want in any amount you want, you may miss out on the many things right before your eyes. I embrace my daily moments without that grip of processed foods. I'd like that outcome for you too—so you can truly be free.

I don't know where your calling is or even if you're living your life with purpose, but what I do know is the answer is waiting within you—the answer for you is in you. Become still and you will hear what you need to hear. And you will see what you need to see. And you will feel what you need to feel. *The answer my friend is in you…*

Acknowledgments

This book represents a personal inquiry into a confusing aspect of my own experience. As I began to make sense out of unexpected changes in my own life, patients with the same needs emerged. This ultimately led to my writing about my discoveries, to share with others in similar situations.

No book is written without the contributions of many people. My wish is to recognize every spoken and unspoken inspired word, but I don't have enough pages, so regrettably I can only mention a few.

I wouldn't have written about these things if not for my husband, Joe, who encourages me to follow my dreams no matter how small or how large they may be. Also, I thank my sons, Kris and Benjamin, who have always been a source of help with technical, legal, and administrative tasks beyond my comprehension. And I must mention with gratitude my beloved parents, Benjamin and Joan, who shine down from heaven, prompting me to continue to move forward in my efforts to help those with similar challenges to the ones I faced.

No book can sing without a great editor, which goes without saying. My editor, G. Miki Hayden, is a godsend. She miraculously breathes life into this mission of mine to help others make peace with the cheat days—food fest frenzy—within many of us.

Last, a huge shout-out to ALL my patients over the past twenty-three years, who taught and continue to teach me. Thank you from my heart!

Bibliography

Bach, D. (1999). *Smart Women Finish Rich.* New York: Broadway Books.

Berkley Media Studies Group. (2011). *The New Age of Marketing: How Companies are Targeting and Luring Our Kids—And What Advocates Can Do About It.* Retrieved on July 1, 2019 from https://bit.ly/2RLUVfn.

Carlson, R. (1997). *Don't Sweat the Small Stuff…and It's All Small Stuff.* New York: Hyperion.

Carlson, R. (1998). *Don't Worry, Make Money: Spiritual and Practical Ways to Create Abundance and More Fun in Your Life.* New York: Hyperion.

Collier, R. (1976). *Riches Within Your Reach: The Law of the Higher Potential.* Ramsey, New
Jersey: Robert Collier Book Corporation.

Collier, R. (2013). *The Secret of the Ages.* New York: Robert Collier Publications, Inc.

DesMaisons, K. (1998). *Potatoes Not Prozac.* New York: Simon & Schuster

Dominguez, J. & Robin, V. (1992). *Your Money or Your Life: Transforming Relationship with Money and Achieving Financial Independence.* New York: Viking.

Dyer, W. (1976). *Your Erroneous Zones: Step-by-Step Advice for Escaping the Trap of Negative Thinking and Taking Control of Your Life*. New York: Funk & Wagnalls.

Dyer, W. (2009). *Excuses Begone!: How to Change Lifelong, Self-Defeating Thinking Habits.* Carlsbad, Ca.: Hay House Publishers.

Dyer, W. (2011). https://www.drwaynedyer.com/blog/tag/excuses-begone/. Retrieved on June, 24, 2019 from Dr. Wayne W. Dyer's Blog.

Dyer, S. and Dyer. W. (2014) *Don't Die with Your Music Still in You: My Experience Growing Up with Spiritual Parents.* Carlsbad, Ca.: Hay House Publishers.

Harvard Women's Health Watch. (2018). "Food and mood: Is there a connection?" Retrieved on May 11, 2019 from: https://www.health.harvard.edu/mind-and-mood/food-and-mood-is-there-a-connection.

Hesse, H. (1998). *Siddhartha.* Mineola, New York: Dover Publications, Inc.

Hill, N. (1983). *Think and Grow Rich.* New York: Ballantine Books.

Johnson, C. (2019). *131 Method.* New York: Hay House, Inc.

Kubler-Ross, E. (1969). *Death and Dying.* New York: Macmillan Publishing Co. Inc.

Livingston, G. (2015). *Never Binge Again: Reprogram Yourself to Think Like a Permanently Thin Person*. Psy Tech Inc.

Livingston, G. (2019). *Psychology Today*: "How to Stop Binge Eating in Three Unusual Steps: A Weird But Systematic Way to Stop Overeating and Binge Eating." Retrieved June 25, 2019 from http://bit.ly/2rrG6WE

Miklas, M. (2012). *Memoirs of a Solo Traveler: My Love Affair with Italy*. United States: Margie Miklas

Ortigara Crego, L. (2017). *Release Your Obsession with Food: Heal from the Inside Out.* Hollywood, Florida: Madeira Publishing.

Ortigara Crego, L. (2018). *Release Your Obsession with Diet Chatter: Heal from the Inside Out.* Hollywood, Florida: Madeira Publishing.

Parsons, H. (1994). *Father Peter Rookey: Man of Miracles.* Australia: Divine Mercy Publications

Pencalski, J. (2019). "The Importance of Family Mealtime." Retrieved on July 31, 2019 from: The Family & Children Center Blog: http://bit.ly/35diSCb

Polcastro, R. (2017). *Death by Gluten: How Undiagnosed Celiac Almost Cost Me My Life.* International: Raw Words Press

Ramsey, D. (2003). *The Total Money Makeover: A Proven Plan for Financial Fitness.* Nashville, Tennessee: Thomas Nelson, Inc.

Ryan, S. (2017). *Simply Keto: A Practical Approach to Health and Weight Loss with 100+ Easy Low Carb Recipes.* Canada: Victory Belt Publishing Inc.

Sanfilipo, D. (2019). *Keto Quick Start: A Beginners Guide to a Whole-Food Ketogenic Diet.* Las Vegas: Victory Belt Publishing Inc.

Sachin, H.J. "Sometimes Food Is the Best Medicine." Retrieved on March 13, 2019 from: http://bit.ly/357sfTP.

Sheppard, K. (2000). *From the First Bite: A Complete Guide to Recovery from Food Addiction.* Deerfield Beach, Fl: Health Communications, Inc.

Sing, M. (2014). "Food, Mood, and Obesity. Frontiers in Psychology." Retrieved on May 13, 2019 from: http://bit.ly/36na64D

Somer, E. (1995). *Food and Mood: The Complete Guide to Eating Well and Feeling Your Best.* New York: Henry Hold and Company, Inc.

Somer, E. (2009). *Eat Your Way to Happiness: 10 Diet Secrets to: Improve Your Mood, Curb Your Cravings, Keep the Pounds Off.* Ontario, Canada: Harlequin.

Stanley, T. & Danko, W. (1996). *The Millionaire Next Door: The Surprising Secrets of America's Wealthy*. Atlanta, Georgia: Longstreet Press.

Vogel, L. (2017). *The Keto Diet: The Complete Guide to a High-Fat Diet.* Canada: Victory Belt Publishing Inc.

About the Author

Dr. Ortigara Crego, a clinical psychotherapist, addiction psychologist, and visiting professor in private practice, has worked in the field of eating disorders for well over two and a half decades. She earned a doctorate in addiction psychology and a Master's degree in social work with the emphasis on mental health, and is certified as an eating disorder specialist, Master's certified addiction professional, and national board-certified clinical hypnotherapist.

Dr. Ortigara Crego worked in the weight-loss industry for well over two decades. She speaks and blogs on recovery from compulsive eating using spiritual and mind approaches to healing. She is the author of *Release Your Obsession with Food: Heal from the Inside Out*, a groundbreaking book on recovering from compulsive eating and spiritual deficits and *Release Your Obsession with Diet Chatter: Heal from the Inside Out*, a much needed book on quieting the drunken monkeys once and for all. She contributed several chapters to SAGE Publications' Volume 1 and Volume 2 of the *Encyclopedia of Obesity* and runs a blog at Weightcontroltherapy.com.

Dr. Ortigara Crego's professional affiliations include the National Association of Social Workers, the National Board for Certified Clinical Hypnotherapists, the International Association of Eating Disorder Professionals, and the American Psychological Association.

Stay in Touch!

Please contact me at drlisaort@weightcontroltherapy.com. I would love to hear from you and learn from your experiences. Stop by my website: http://weightcontroltherapy.com. to see what I'm up to and where I'm speaking next, along with what books I have planned, such as the next in the Release Your Obsession series, *Release Your Obsession with Ageing: Heal from the Inside Out.*

You can also find me on:
Facebook (www.facebook.com/Drlisaortigaracrego)
Twitter: (www.twitter.com/Drlisort)
Instagram: (www.Instagram.com/Drlisaort)

Where we can exchange lively discussions on topics of health, including mental, physical, and spiritual wellbeing.

Thank you for reading *Release Your Obsession with Cheat DAZE: Heal from the Inside Out.* If you found it informative and helpful and have the inclination, please consider writing a review for the author on Amazon.com, Goodreads and Barnes and Noble. It really does make a difference.

Also by Dr. Lisa Ortigara Crego

Release Your Obsession with Food: Heal from the Inside Out

Release Your Obsession with Diet Chatter: Heal from the Inside Out

Weekly Blog found on www.weightcontroltherapy.com

Made in the USA
Monee, IL
08 November 2026

68156251R00194